Ethics Consultation

Ethics Consultation • From Theory to Practice

Edited by MARK P. AULISIO, PH.D.

ROBERT M. ARNOLD, M.D.

and STUART J. YOUNGNER, M.D.

The Johns Hopkins University Press

BALTIMORE AND LONDON

© 2003 The Johns Hopkins University Press
All rights reserved. Published 2003
Printed in the United States of America on acid-free paper

9 8 7 6 5 4 3 2 1

The Johns Hopkins University Press
2715 North Charles Street
Baltimore, Maryland 21218-4363
www.press.jhu.edu

Library of Congress Cataloging-in-Publication Data
Ethics consultation : from theory to practice / edited by Mark P.
Aulisio, Robert M. Arnold, and Stuart J. Youngner.
   p.   cm.
Includes bibliographical references and index.
ISBN 0-8018-7165-4
1. Medical ethics consultation. I. Aulisio, Mark P., 1965– II.
Arnold, Robert M., 1957– III. Youngner, Stuart J.
R724 .E821112 2003
174'.2—dc21
2002006241

A catalog record for this book is available from the British Library.

Contents

5. Techniques for Training Ethics Consultants: Why Traditional Classroom Methods Are Not Enough

6. Models for Ethics Consultation: Individual, Team, or Committee?

7. The Structure and Process of Ethics Consultation Services

8. Institutional Support for Bioethics Committees

Contributors

Robert M. Arnold, M.D., is Professor and Leo H. Criep Chair in Patient Care in the Department of Medicine at the University of Pittsburgh School of Medicine, Associate Director for Education at the Center for Bioethics and Health Law, and Chief of the Section of Palliative Care and Medical Ethics.

Mark P. Aulisio, Ph.D., is Director of the Clinical Ethics Program at Metro-Health Medical Center and Assistant Professor of Bioethics in the Department of Bioethics at Case Western Reserve University School of Medicine.

Françoise Baylis, Ph.D., is Professor in the Department of Bioethics in the Faculty of Medicine at Dalhousie University, with a cross-appointment in the Department of Philosophy.

Charles Bosk, Ph.D., is Professor in the Department of Sociology and the Center for Bioethics at the University of Pennsylvania.

Dan W. Brock, Ph.D., is Senior Scientist in the Department of Clinical Bioethics at the National Institutes of Health, and Charles C. Tillinghast, Jr., University Professor Emeritus of Philosophy and Biomedical Ethics at Brown University.

Howard Brody, M.D., Ph.D., is Professor of Family Practice and Philosophy and has an appointment in the Center for Ethics and Humanities in the Life Sciences at Michigan State University.

Linda L. Emanuel, M.D., Ph.D., is Buehler Professor of Medicine, Director of the Buehler Center on Aging, and Director of the Interdisciplinary Program in Professionalism and Human Rights at Northwestern University Medical School.

John C. Fletcher, Ph.D., is Professor Emeritus of Biomedical Ethics and Internal Medicine at University of Virginia School of Medicine.

Jacqueline J. Glover, Ph.D., is Associate Professor of Medicine and Pediatrics and Associate Director of the Center for Health Ethics and Law at West Virginia University.

Steven Miles, M.D., is Associate Professor in the Department of Medicine and the Center for Biomedical Ethics at the University of Minnesota.

Jonathan Moreno, Ph.D., is Kornfeld Professor and Director of the Center for Biomedical Ethics and Professor of Medical Education in the Department of Health Evaluation Sciences at the University of Virginia.

Kathryn L. Moseley, M.D., is Director of Biomedical Ethics for the Henry Ford Health System.

William Nelson, Ph.D., is Education Coordinator at the National Center for Ethics in Health Care, Veterans Health Administration. He is also Adjunct Associate Professor of Community and Family Medicine at Dartmouth Medical School and Adjunct Associate Professor of Psychiatry at New York University School of Medicine.

Ruth B. Purtilo, Ph.D., is Director and Dr. C. C. and Mabel L. Criss Professor of Clinical Ethics at Creighton University Center for Health Policy and Ethics.

Cynda Rushton, M.S.N., D.N.Sc., is Assistant Professor of Nursing and on the faculty of the Bioethics Institute, The Johns Hopkins University, and is Clinical Nurse Specialist in Ethics and Project Director of the Harriet Lane Compassionate Care Program at The Johns Hopkins Children's Center.

Paul M. Schyve, M.D., is Senior Vice President of the Joint Commission on Accreditation of Healthcare Organizations.

Melanie H. Wilson Silver, Ph.D., is a Health Care Ethics Consultant based in southern New Jersey. She consults and teaches in both the United States and England.

Joy Skeel, M.Div., B.S.N., is Director of the Ethics Consultation Service and Professor of Medical Humanities and Ethics at the Medical College of Ohio.

William Winslade, J.D., Ph.D., is James Wade Rockwell Professor of Philosophy of Medicine at the Institute for the Medical Humanities, University of Texas Medical Branch.

Stuart J. Youngner, M.D., is Chairman of the Department of Bioethics and Susan B. Watson Professor of Bioethics and Professor of Psychiatry at Case Western Reserve University School of Medicine.

Preface

Mr. Jones, an 82-year-old man, came to the emergency room with a gangrenous leg. He had fallen in his apartment and was unable to contact family or friends. He was discovered by his niece, his closest living relative, two days later. Mr. Jones, who was otherwise healthy, needed to have his leg amputated in order to save his life. (Without amputation, he was likely to die from septicemia.) He adamantly refused amputation and expressed a deep desire to die "in one piece." Mr. Jones's niece was devastated by his refusal of amputation and wanted the health care team to save her uncle's life. She felt responsible for his condition, since she was supposed to check in on him every day, but she had missed a day due to illness. Members of the health care team were split over whether Mr. Jones's refusal of treatment should be honored. The attending physician believed that the team had a moral obligation to go ahead with amputation, since it was a "straightforward, relatively low risk procedure that could save Mr. Jones's life." He argued that the procedure was "ordinary," not "extraordinary," and therefore obligatory. He emphatically stated, "I became a doctor to save life, not to watch people die because they are afraid!" Other members of the health care team, especially several nurses, thought Mr. Jones's wishes should be respected. Some worried, however, that Mr. Jones might be depressed and was trying to kill himself by refusing amputation.[1]

The case of Mr. Jones is complex and multifaceted, layered with medical, psychosocial, legal, and ethical dimensions. Mr. Jones, his niece, the attending physician, and members of the nursing staff all have different views of what should be done, but they are at an impasse. What should be done, and why? The case of Mr. Jones is representative of the types of cases that have been discussed in bioethics over the years, and these cases can be and, of course, are being dealt with in a variety of contexts.

One context is that of academe. In the classroom setting, the case of Mr. Jones might be looked at from the standpoint of orthodox Roman Catholic moral theology, orthodox Judaism, act or rule utilitarianism, Kantian "respect for persons," or any one of a number of other theoretical perspectives. In the comfort of academe, the case of Mr. Jones might be situated in a variety of social and political contexts as well (that of a minimal state or of a welfare state, and so on). This attests to the richness of bioethical issues and the corresponding richness of academic discussion.

The case of Mr. Jones, though a rich source for academic speculation, is also typical of cases that come before ethics committees and consultants. In the clinical context of ethics consultation, such cases are anything but academic. The clinical context is multidisciplinary, multiperspectival, and, quite unlike that of the academy, driven by a time-pressured practical need to move forward in decision making. In the clinical context of ethics consultation, these cases raise a host of questions, both theoretical and practical:

Is there really a need for ethics consultation in contemporary health care?

If so, is there any legitimate approach to meeting that need that is consistent with the basic societal values of our liberal democracy?

What kinds of education and training, knowledge and skills, should ethics committee members or consultants have?

If ethics consultation is to be done at all, is it best done by individual consultants, small teams, full ethics committees, or some combination of these?

What kinds of structures and processes should be followed as an ethics consultation is carried out?

Do institutions have an obligation to support ethics mechanisms, and, if so, what types of support should be offered?

Should those who do ethics consultation be licensed, certified, or otherwise accredited?

These types of questions motivated the development of the American Society for Bioethics and Humanities (ASBH) Task Force on Standards for Bioethics Consultation back in 1995; comprised the report of that task force, *Core Competencies for Health Care Ethics Consultation* (hereafter referred to as the ASBH report; see Appendix for the full report), published three years later; and form the focus of this volume, which draws its impetus from the ASBH report.[2]

Real clinical cases that come before consultants or committees come with a rich context already provided, with multiple players and perspectives, and with a practical need for resolution. Indeed, practical issues form the heart of this volume: issues such as whether ethics consultation is best done by individuals, teams, or committees (Chapter 6), how an ethics consultation service should be structured and the appropriate processes for carrying out consultations (Chapter 7), the need for institutional support of such services (Chapter 8), and

techniques and programs for educating and training those who staff consultation services (Chapters 4 and 5). Even where the volume takes a theoretical
turn, as in addressing a proper approach to ethics consultation (Chapters 1 and
2) or the importance of character (Chapter 3), or a speculative turn, as in
addressing questions on the horizon for ethics consultants, such as organizational ethics (Chapter 9) or professionalization and certification (Chapter 10),
the theoretical and speculative discussion is aimed at the "real-world" practice
of ethics consultation. Indeed, all the issues addressed herein stem from questions and controversies dealt with as the Task Force on Standards for Bioethics
Consultation struggled to develop its report on ethics consultation, a report
focused on the competencies necessary to *do* health care ethics consultation.
We hope, therefore, that this volume will be both interesting and useful to a
broad spectrum of the bioethics community, ranging from academic bioethicists to health professionals on the front lines, sitting on ethics committees and
doing consultation.

Part I, "Foundational and Theoretical Questions," focuses on several questions that must be addressed before the more practical issues of Part II can be
taken up. First, Chapters 1 and 2 tackle such basic questions as whether there is a
need for ethics consultation in health care today, and, if so, what approach best
meets that need while remaining consistent with fundamental societal values.
Chapter 3 addresses an issue that was both difficult and controversial in task
force deliberations: the relationship between the character of consultants and
the role of ethics consultation. Should there be character requirements for
ethics consultants that extend beyond behavior exhibited in ethics consultation? Should consultants view themselves, or encourage others to view them, as
role models of good character or virtue? The chapter, like the task force itself, is divided on this topic. Answers to these questions affect a number of
other issues, ranging from the selection of ethics consultants to their education
and training.

In Chapter 1, "Meeting the Need: Ethics Consultation in Health Care Today,"
Mark P. Aulisio takes up the task of laying the justificatory foundation for the
"ethics facilitation" approach to ethics consultation endorsed in the ASBH
report. He does this by showing (1) how the need for ethics consultation arises
in our society (technological advancement, the social fact of pluralism, the
political rights of individuals to live by their own conception of the good life,
etc.), (2) why what the ASBH report terms "authoritarian" and "pure facilitation" approaches fail to meet that need, and (3) why the "ethics facilitation"
approach as described in the report both is justified in our societal context

and addresses the need for ethics consultation that arises from that context. Dr. Aulisio employs a series of cases, actual and hypothetical, to illustrate the need for ethics consultation in contemporary health care settings and to show the relevant features of the context that help to define a proper role for it.

Jonathan Moreno, in Chapter 2, "Can Ethics Consultation Be Saved? Ethics Consultation and Moral Consensus in a Democratic Society," elaborates a theory of moral consensus in a democratic society and assesses the ASBH report, and in particular the conception of ethics consultation it articulates, in the light of that theory. Interestingly, while he takes a different tack from that of the report, his view of the role of ethics consultation turns out to be very similar. Moral consensus, according to Dr. Moreno, should be viewed as a process rather than an event. The standards that should govern moral consensus will, therefore, be process standards. Dr. Moreno then argues that, from an ethical standpoint, these process standards should embody certain liberal, democratic values in a society such as ours. Among these values will be an openness to alternative points of view, for example. Thus, if ethics consultation is to be seen as an aid in achieving a satisfactory moral consensus, it will, in Dr. Moreno's view, have to serve those values.

The final chapter of this part takes up an issue that was a flashpoint of considerable controversy in task force deliberations: the relationship between good character or virtue and ethics consultation. In keeping with the division in the task force on this issue, Chapter 3 features two distinct views (pro and con) of character requirements for those who do ethics consultation. In the section "The Importance of Character for Health Care Ethics Consultation," Françoise Baylis and Howard Brody argue that character is centrally important to the role ethics consultants should play in health care settings. They argue that good character or virtue is more central to the role of being an ethics consultant than it is to the roles played by health professionals—so much so, they argue, that consultants should be role models of virtue for others. To be sure, Drs. Baylis and Brody do not suggest, and indeed they explicitly reject, that this means any particular ethics consultant, or even ethics consultants in general, are more virtuous than others in health care; they are simply suggesting that good character or virtue is more central to the ethics consultant's role. In the section "Whose Virtue? Which Character?" Mark P. Aulisio, Dan Brock, and William Winslade take a very different tack. After pointing out some of the vexed problems inherent in discussions of "character" or "virtue," such as profound definitional issues, they argue that expanding the ethics consultant's role to include being a role model or exemplar of virtue, as Baylis and Brody do, begs for an answer to the questions "Whose virtue? Which character?"—and in so doing threatens to undermine the role for ethics consultation laid out in the ASBH report itself.

Part II, "Practical Questions," which is composed of Chapters 4 through 8 and forms the heart of this volume, has a very practical bent. Chapters 4 and 5 focus on education and training of consultants, while Chapters 6, 7, and 8 discuss basic functional issues such as whether ethics consultation should be done by individuals, teams, or committees; how ethics consultation services might be structured; and the obligations of institutions to support consultation services.

In Chapter 4, "Innovative Educational Programs: A Necessary First Step toward Improving Quality in Ethics Consultation," Jacqueline J. Glover and William Nelson address the importance of education and training for those who do ethics consultation. While the chapter does not intend to be exhaustive, it highlights several innovative continuing education programs in ethics that are directed to health professionals who are engaged in ethics consultation, education, and/or policy formation in their institutions but cannot pursue an advanced degree in bioethics. This group constitutes the overwhelming majority of those who do ethics consultation, while remaining the most underserved. Drs. Glover and Nelson devote particular attention to how these programs address the core competencies for ethics consultation outlined in the ASBH report. Various evaluation strategies used in connection with these programs are also discussed.

In Chapter 5, "Techniques for Training Ethics Consultants: Why Traditional Classroom Methods Are Not Enough," Robert M. Arnold and Melanie H. Wilson Silver tackle the issue of how to train ethics consultants so that they acquire the relevant knowledge and skills. This issue is especially pressing for process and interpersonal skills, which the ASBH report emphasizes as being acquired mainly through "hands on" experience, or "doing." Drs. Arnold and Wilson Silver suggest that traditional classroom methods will not be adequate for imparting some of these skills. This chapter outlines some alternative training techniques, such as role-plays and mock consultations, for developing relevant skills and knowledge. Three issues, however, remain unresolved: (1) how to evaluate whether consultants possess these skills, and the relationship between such skills and "good" consultation; (2) the impact of requiring these skills on the composition of teams of ethics consultants (as only social workers receive much of the facilitative training discussed in the chapter); and (3) whether small hospitals will devote the resources necessary to train professionals in this way. (The divergence between Chapters 4 and 5 is telling in this regard.)

In Chapter 6, "Models for Ethics Consultation: Individual, Team, or Committee?" Cynda Rushton, Stuart J. Youngner, and Joy Skeel deal with one of the more important practical issues raised by the work of the task force: whether the individual, team, or committee model (or some hybrid of these) is most effective for ethics consultation. Though the task force explicitly stated that it was not taking a position on this question, further exploration of this practical issue is warranted. Professors Rushton, Youngner, and Skeel consider the strengths and weaknesses of each type of model, offer suggestions for enhancing the effectiveness of each, and endorse the small-team model as optimal for most consultations. The small-team model, they argue, captures the relevant strengths of both individual and committee models, while avoiding some of their most salient drawbacks.

In Chapter 7, "The Structure and Process of Ethics Consultation Services," John C. Fletcher and Kathryn L. Moseley deal with the tangled process questions that confront ethics consultation services, including:

Who should know about the existence and modus operandi of the ethics consultation service?

How should they be informed?

Who should be informed that an ethics consultation is taking place?

Who should be able to make a request or block a request for an ethics consultation?

Who should participate in an ethics consultation, and to what degree?

Who should be informed about the results of an ethics consultation, and in what manner?

This chapter explores these important questions in detail, giving a taxonomy of the "process" and "structural" issues raised by consultation. In so doing, Drs. Fletcher and Moseley offer an interesting discussion of six legal cases in which ethics consultants have been named or criticized and point out process elements that contributed to the cause in each suit. They argue that there are certain normative requirements for the structure of ethics consultation services that all such services should meet, while remaining sensitive to the specific circumstances and culture of different health care institutions.

In the final chapter of this part, Chapter 8, "Institutional Support for Bioethics Committees," Steven Miles and Ruth B . Purtilo explore why health care institutions should provide resources to their ethics services. The basic premise of the ASBH report is that certain skills and knowledge are required for ethics consultation. Drs. Miles and Purtilo point out that developing, retaining, and improving such skill and knowledge requires support. They elaborate on the types of resources needed (e.g., time, libraries, association memberships, tuition support); explain how and why health care institutions should foster a climate in which those performing ethics consultations can work with integrity and what that climate would be like; and show how this support is related to quality assurance. Drs. Miles and Purtilo emphasize the basic fact that without institutional support, the obligation of quality assurance and improvement in ethics consultation, as in other clinical services, will inevitably go unsatisfied.

In Part III, "Questions on the Horizon," the concluding chapters take a forward-looking view in trying to assess what might be on the horizon for ethics consultation and those who have the responsibility for carrying it out. Should we expect a greater role for organizational ethics consultation as the boundaries between the bedside and the boardroom continue to blur (Chapter 9)? Will ethics consultants face increasing pressure to move ever closer to professionalization, would this be a good or a bad thing, and under what circumstances, if any, might it be appropriate for ethics consultants to have to satisfy a certification or licensure process (Chapter 10)?

In Chapter 9, "Organizational Ethics: Promises and Pitfalls," Paul M. Schyve, Linda L. Emanuel, William Winslade, and Stuart J. Youngner look at this rapidly developing domain for ethics consultation (spurred on by pressures stemming from market-driven medicine and the emergence of managed care, as well as from the Joint Commission on the Accreditation of Healthcare Organizations and the Office of the Inspector General). Organizational ethics, they argue, poses special challenges because it involves the intersection of three historically disparate ethical traditions: those of the bedside, the boardroom, and the community. This chapter looks at the kinds of issues that are emerging under the umbrella of "organizational ethics" and suggests the types of competencies that should be embodied in ethics committees that deal with them. The question of whether institutions should have separate committees to deal with "organizational" and "clinical" issues is also considered, as is the appropriateness of the "ethics facilitation" approach, as advocated in the ASBH report, for organizational ethics consultation.

Fittingly, this volume concludes, like the ASBH report itself, by revisiting the controversial issues of professionalization, certification, and licensure, in Chapter 10, "The Licensing and Certification of Ethics Consultants: What Part of "No!" Was So Hard to Understand?" by Charles Bosk. The ASBH report recommended that standards for ethics consultation be voluntary "at this time," while rejecting certification. This does not, of course, imply that the task force contemplated more stringent, mandatory guidelines at some later time. Nonetheless, this question does not promise to go away anytime soon. What, then, are the future developments that would cause a revisiting and a revision of optional guidelines? What future developments would induce more prescriptive certainty about standards for ethics consultation? Dr. Bosk discusses the merits and demerits of certification and licensure, while identifying some of the developments that might make such credentialing appropriate, or even necessary, for ethics consultants at some point in the future. Indeed, this chapter is especially timely in that even as this book goes to press, the issue of credentialing for ethics consultants remains controversial and is again being taken up by a committee of the ASBH.

As you move through each chapter of this volume, we ask that you not allow us to take you too far afield from that originating context of clinical bioethics, with its many layers, players, and perspectives and its practical need for resolution. We ask you to think back periodically on the case of Mr. Jones and other real cases from your own experience and to consider what kind of approach to ethics consultation these real cases warrant. We ask you to consider the issues raised and how they might best be addressed. We ask you to consider the kinds of skills, knowledge, and/or character traits that those engaged in addressing these issues might need, and how such skills, knowledge, and/or character traits might be acquired. In short, we ask that you not allow us to make this a purely academic discussion, but rather relate it to your own experience so that the very real needs of Mr. Jones, his niece, members of the care team, and others like them do not go unmet.

Notes

1. Aulisio, M.P., "Ethics Consultation: Is It Enough to Mean Well?" *HEC Forum* 11, no. 3 (1999):208–17.

2. This task force was convened prior to the development of the American Society for Bioethics and Humanities and was sponsored by the Society for Health and Human Values (SHHV) and the Society for Bioethics Consultation (SBC). Thus, the task force was the SHHV-SBC Task Force on Standards for Bioethics Consultation. These organi-

zations later merged with the American Association of Bioethics (AAB) to form the ASBH. The ASBH adopted the SHHV-SBC Task Force report. In order to avoid confusion, we will refer to this task force as the ASBH Task Force on Standards for Bioethics Consultation. For further detail on origins, please see "I. Introduction" of the task force report which is reproduced as an appendix to this volume.

I • FOUNDATIONAL AND THEORETICAL QUESTIONS

1

Meeting the Need

Ethics Consultation in Health Care Today

MARK P. AULISIO, PH.D.

THE CASE OF THE BELOVED BROTHER: "I KNOW WHY YOU'RE HERE"

A 72-year-old white male was admitted to the SICU [surgical intensive care unit] for a ruptured aortic aneurysm. Although he initially did well and was discharged to a long-term care facility, he was soon readmitted for a massive GI bleed. He underwent surgery but unfortunately re-bled, resulting in cerebral ischemia with mental status changes. He became ventilator dependent, developed renal and liver failure, and sepsis. He was placed on dialysis.

The patient had a sister and a brother, with both of whom he was very close. The sister was the recognized decision maker in the family. She insisted on aggressive therapy and wanted "everything done." Aggressive therapy was instituted and continued for about three weeks without any improvement in status. After three weeks, the nursing staff felt that aggressive treatment was inappropriate and that the patient did not want it. They reported that the patient periodically grimaced when turned and suctioned. One nurse reported that before intubation the patient said, "Why are you doing this to me? I've had enough. I'm dying, aren't I?" Also, the nursing staff relayed that the patient's brother said that the patient was angry that he was readmitted (and intubated). The nursing staff did not initially oppose aggressive therapy because they thought the sister "needed time" and would "come around." The SICU attending now agrees with the nursing staff that continued aggressive therapy is inappropriate. They would like to stop dialysis. The patient's sister remains adamant that "everything be done."

The head nurse called for an ethics consultation because her staff "cannot continue to do this to that poor man." They are angry and upset with the patient's sister. The ethics consultation team, after meeting with the attending and the nursing staff, set up a meeting with the patient's sister and brother. The patient's sister starts the meeting with the consultation team by saying, "I know why you're here. They want you to convince me to give up on my brother [she starts to cry], but you don't understand . . . I can never give up on my brother [sobbing] . . . How could you ask me to give up on my brother? How could I live with myself if I gave up on him? I love him so much [her brother comforts her]."[1]

Over the past thirty years, ethics consultation has become increasingly common in clinical settings. Indeed, a recent study indicated that 100% of U.S. hospitals with 400 beds or more, federal hospitals, or hospitals that are members of the Council of Teaching Hospitals and over 81% of all U.S. hospitals now have an ethics consultation service of some kind.[2] There is no question that the development of ethics mechanisms in health care (usually an ethics committee) has been spurred by several landmark court cases and encouraged by the Joint Commission on Accreditation of Healthcare Organizations (JCAHO).[3] Historically, however, ethics consultation has been the least utilized and most controversial function of an ethics committee, taking a backseat to education and policy formation.

The controversy surrounding ethics consultation has stemmed from disputes about whether it has an appropriate role in contemporary health care settings. Some have suggested that there is no need for ethics consultation, since doctors, nurses, and other health professionals can and should handle ethical issues as they arise. Others have more forcefully criticized ethics consultation as at odds with the fundamental values of a democratic society, a society in which no particular moral view should be privileged (the idea that "when it comes to ethics, either all are experts or none are").[4] Though there are strands of truth in both claims, neither matches the poignancy or rhetorical force of the patient's sister in the case above: "I know why you're here. They want you to convince me to give up on my brother"—a powerful, embarrassing, and honest insinuation of illegitimacy.

In this chapter, I tackle this fundamental question for ethics consultation: does it have a legitimate place in contemporary health care? To do so, I look at whether there is a need for ethics consultation in health care today and, if so, what approach to ethics consultation, if any, best meets that need while remaining consistent with the fundamental values of our society. I argue that certain salient contextual features of health care today, fundamental societal values foremost among them, create a need for ethics consultation and therefore must inform an appropriate approach to meeting that need. Ultimately, I argue that the "ethics facilitation" approach characterized in *Core Competencies for Health Care Ethics Consultation: The Report of the American Society for Bioethics and Humanities* (the ASBH report) charts an appropriate mean between two illegitimate extremes in being informed by and responding to the need for ethics consultation in contemporary health care.

Is There a Need?

Whether there is a need for ethics consultation in health care today is, as we have seen, a matter of some dispute. The proliferation of ethics consultation services in recent years, though suggestive of need, does not establish it. Historically, the doctor-patient relationship formed the locus of decision making, and some would argue that medical practice was done quite well without such outside intrusions as ethics committees and consultation services. Just how well medicine was practiced in the past is debatable, of course, but I suggest that at least three salient features of health care today converge to create the need for ethics consultation: complexity of decision making, value heterogeneity, and a growing recognition of the rights of individuals and the implications of those rights for health care.

Complexity of Decision Making

Thanks to the pace of technological developments, health care today is more complex than ever. We are faced with choices that were unimaginable just a few decades ago. Decisions about whether to withdraw ventilator support, administer food and hydration through a central line, or perform dialysis simply did not have to be made prior to the emergence of modern medicine and more recent advances in technology.

Even as the complexity and number of choices facing patients, families, and providers multiplies, the contemporary health care environment is increasingly less conducive to good decision making. In acute care settings, for example, delivery of care is divided along service lines that often fail to communicate well with one another or that send mixed messages to patients, families, and surrogates. Partly due to the rise of managed care, doctors spend less time with their patients, and patients have shorter and less well-established relationships with their primary care physicians. Economic considerations drive decision making perhaps more powerfully, and certainly more overtly, than in the past, and greater attention is being paid to balancing the needs of the one against the good of the many.

Though the complexity of medical decision making today may create a greater need for doctors and other health professionals to spend more time with patients, and for patients to be more actively involved in their care, it does not by itself create a need for ethics consultation. Rather, today's complex medical decision making goes on in a broader societal context of value heterogeneity and a growing recognition of the implications of individual rights for that decision making, which combine with the current clinical reality to create the need for ethics consultation.

Value Heterogeneity

THE CAVE CASE: "WE JUST DON'T AGREE"

One bright sunny day, you and five of your friends decide to go spelunking. You are relatively inexperienced and unprepared spelunkers (as most of us are), but, undeterred, you boldly head off into the caves of a nearby state park. After a few hours trekking into the bowels of the caves you feel a tremor, and then, suddenly, a cave-in crashes down just behind you, leaving you and your friends trapped and afraid. After a time, you and your friends regain your composure and endeavor to find a way out. You journey on for several more hours, and to the great joy and relief of all, you spy daylight in the distance. The group rushes ahead toward the narrow escape, when again there is a sudden tremor, which hurls the largest member of your party into the narrow escape, lodging him inextricably. At the same time, the tremor precipitates another cave-in—again, just behind your group. You and your friends are now stuck in the small space that remains, behind your unfortunate companion who is lodged in the sole narrow escape from your dark, damp, cold prison. You push and pull—try to dig under and around him—but to no avail. As luck would have it, one of your friends has a small explosive, which would not be enough to blow a hole through the thick rocky front sides of the cave but would be more than adequate to blow your companion out of the narrow mouth. Oxygen is in short supply. You are beginning to feel faint, and, behind you, the cave slowly begins to fill with water.[5]

Paternalistic medicine was feasible in an era when doctors and patients were faced with comparatively few choices and shared similar values about medical care. Doctors' and patients' values sometimes differed, of course, but even this could be offset by the presence of a longstanding relationship and a characteristic cultural deference to physicians' authority.[6] Today, however, our society is increasingly pluralistic in its values, and the health care arena is no exception.

When I discuss the relevance of ethics for clinical practice with groups of health professionals, I like to stimulate discussion by starting with the above variation on Lon Fuller's famous case of the Speluncean Explorers, which has the ignoble and impolitic title "The Fat Man in the Cave." The standard array of responses is given by almost every group. The kinder, gentler types insist they would try every possible way to free the unfortunate man, all without hurting him. Of course, since the whole point of the case is to push people to explore their moral intuitions about whether it might be acceptable, praiseworthy, or required to kill the one so that the many (five) might live, I don't allow these standard practical maneuvers to succeed. After the distinction between "would," "could," and "should" is clarified (as there are always some who will agree that the one must die that the many might live, but see themselves as psychologically incapable of killing the poor chap), most groups divide about evenly on what the morally appropriate course of action might be. The standard moves of justification and excuse (e.g., self-defense) are usually forthcoming as well.

What is interesting about the exercise for our purposes, however, is the broad range of moral views brought forward by discussants. Though not explicitly labeled as such by participants, the views expressed cross the moral spectrum to include, among others, variations on utilitarian, egoist, natural law, rights, and a variety of religious views. Discussants inevitably do not agree on *what* should be done, and those who do agree on *what* should be done often don't agree on *why* it should be done. In short, the Cave exercise invariably shows that, as a society, we have a wide plurality of moral views or, more simply, that we have very different values.

But Who Is Right?

In addition to illustrating the pluralistic nature (value heterogeneity) of contemporary society, the Cave exercise serves to underscore another important feature of the societal context in which health care decision making must go on: there is no particular privileged substantive moral view. Individuals in our society have a right to hold their own moral views—their own values—by which they choose to live.[7] In my experience, when asked "Who is right?" discussants of the Cave case usually, after vigorous debate and failed efforts at suasion, agree that others have a *right* to be wrong. Indeed, irrespective of whether there is a "correct" moral view, individuals in our society have the right to live their lives by their values (within certain limits). We are religious and nonreligious, utilitarians and Kantians, egoists and natural lawyers, atheists and theists, and we have a right to be so. Furthermore, individuals involved in health care retain these rights, whether they are patients, family members, surrogates, or nurses, doctors, and social workers.

Values and Medical Decision Making

The value heterogeneity described above is, not surprisingly, reflected in the clinical context, but it would be of little significance for health care if different individuals' values did not have implications for medical decision making. Individuals' values do, however, have important implications for medical decision making, as the following case illustrates.

THE CASE OF THE MULTITALENTED MOTORCYCLIST: "A MEDICAL NO-BRAINER"?

A patient is brought into the emergency room following a bad motorcycle accident. Due to lack of blood flow, the patient's right leg is in danger. A vein could be taken from the wrist and placed in the leg to save it, leaving the patient with a minor disability in the wrist. The patient insists on having the leg amputated.[8]

This case is, obviously, a thin hypothetical example contrived to illustrate the value-laden nature of medical decision making. It usually elicits a few laughs when presented to groups of health professionals, and a common initial response is to question the patient's *competency*—a reasonable reaction given the apparent oddity of the patient's choice—and her *understanding* of the real options with which she is faced.[9] As the case is explained further, however, the patient is revealed to be both competent and well informed, which makes her choice more perplexing. What might make sense of this peculiar decision?

The case is rigged, of course: it turns out that the patient is a concert pianist, making her choice perfectly understandable. Albeit purposely simplistic and contrived, the case illustrates in a clear and intuitive way the profound implications an individual's values can have for medical decision making. What appeared to be a medically obvious course, saving the patient's leg, turned out to be value-dependent. Given *our* values, most of us would choose to have a minor wrist disability. However, given the pianist *patient's* values, amputation is clearly the "best treatment" for her.[10]

Convergence in the Clinic: The Need for Ethics Consultation

The complexity of technology-driven modern health care, value heterogeneity, individual rights, and the implications of differences in individuals' values for medical decision making—all converge to create a need for ethics consultation in contemporary health care. It is, perhaps, easiest to see the implications of an individual's values for medical decision making when that person is the patient. We must remember, however, that all parties involved in decision making in any given case have their own values as well. When multiple parties who may not share the same values are involved in a complex decision, it is easy to see how value uncertainty or even conflict can arise.[11] The practical need to move forward when this happens presses for a resolution.[12]

Before we turn to the discussion of an appropriate approach to ethics consultation, a clarification is in order. One might object that the factors identified above do not *necessarily* establish a need for *ethics consultation,* but rather simply illustrate how challenging some decisions in contemporary health care settings have become. This objection highlights an important point about the relationship between what I am calling the "need" for ethics consultation and "ethics consultation" itself, a point that should be made explicit. The *practical* need to move forward with decision making is thwarted by the complexity of the decision making itself, and, in particular, normative value conflicts and uncertainties that arise in a context that both is pluralistic and affirms the rights of individuals to live by their values. This, in large part, is the need that "ethics consultation" has emerged to address. Perhaps the need could have come to be addressed in other ways, suggesting a *contingent* rather than a *necessary* connection between "ethics consultation" and the "need." Nonetheless, the need is real and is one that ethics consultation emerged to address. Given this need, then, how should ethics consultation be approached?

Finding an Appropriate Approach to Ethics Consultation

Having highlighted some of the salient factors that give rise to the need for ethics consultation in contemporary health care, we can now return to our original case, the Beloved Brother, to see (1) how those factors play out in creating the need for ethics consultation and (2) how that need might be appropriately addressed. In so doing, we will look at several approaches to ethics consultation characterized in the ASBH report to consider which is most appropriate given the context that creates the need for ethics consultation in the first place.

In the case of the Beloved Brother, all the contextual features highlighted above converge to create the need for ethics consultation. The case, though powerful, is in this respect fairly typical of the kinds of cases that come before consultants and committees. Contemporary medical technology—here, ventilator support and dialysis—creates and drives the choice to continue or discontinue life-sustaining treatment. Involved parties, from caregivers to the patient's sister and brother, ostensibly agree about the facts but disagree about what should be done and why—a largely value-dependent disagreement. Finally, all parties have a right to hold their divergent views. The case is stalemated and the practical need for a resolution is pressing. Thus, we can argue the need for ethics consultation, but how should that need be met? Why *are* we there, anyway?

The ASBH report characterizes two extreme approaches to meeting the need for ethics consultation, *authoritarian* and *pure facilitation,* in order to (1) highlight extremes to be avoided and (2) contrast those extremes with a more appropriate approach to ethics consultation, *ethics facilitation.*[13] We now look at how each of these approaches is characterized in the ASBH report and their implications for our case.[14]

Authoritarian Approach

As characterized in the ASBH report, an *authoritarian* approach to ethics consultation emphasizes "consultants as the primary moral decision makers at the expense of appropriate moral decision makers."[15] The following examples are offered to illustrate two different types of authoritarian approaches, *outcome* and *process.*

To illustrate the inadequacies of an authoritarian approach to the outcome of consultation, consider a case in which a competent well-informed adult patient refuses treatment on religious grounds (suppose the patient is a Jehovah's Witness and the treatment involves blood products). Imagine that the ethics consultant is very sensitive to the process of consultation and talks to the involved parties, addressing the factual, conceptual, and normative issues raised by the case. The consultant then recommends that the patient be given treatment against his wishes, arguing that his religious beliefs are false. As this case illustrates, an authoritarian approach to the outcome of consultation makes the ethics consultant the primary moral decision maker and displaces the appropriate moral decision maker, in this case the patient. This approach places the personal moral values of the ethics consultant over those of the other parties in the case. By misplacing moral decision-making authority, this approach fails to recognize the appropriate boundaries for ethics consultation, as fundamentally established by the rights of individuals in our society.[16]

To illustrate the inadequacies of an authoritarian approach to the process of consultation, consider a case in which a family and health care team disagree over continued treatment of a critically ill adolescent. Suppose the health care team believes continued treatment is futile, while the family hopes for the patient's miraculous recovery. Imagine that the ethics consultant, after talking to the attending physician and reviewing the chart, sides with the health care team and recommends that treatment be discontinued. The consultant does not reach this decision based on personal moral views, but rather from an understanding of the controversial concept of *futility* as discussed in the bio-ethics literature. This approach is authoritarian in its process because it excludes relevant parties from moral decision making. It fails to open lines of communication between the family and the health care team so as to work toward a consensus that falls within the boundaries set by societal values, law, and institutional policy.[17]

Both authoritarian approaches to ethics consultation characterized in the ASBH report, though importantly different, share the key characteristic of focusing on consultants as the primary moral decision makers. In the first case, outcome authoritarianism, ethics consultants take on the role of substantive moral experts, able to adjudicate on the content of an individual's moral values. In the second case, process authoritarianism, consultants, perhaps because they presume a sort of substantive moral expertise, ride roughshod over an inclusive process, excluding key decision makers from the very process of decision making itself. The authoritarian approach as characterized here is, of course, a caricature, but it is instructive as it illustrates some dangers to be avoided—real dangers that come up in actual cases.

These dangers can be seen clearly as we look again at the case of the Beloved Brother. Indeed, the most plausible reading of the sister's words "I know why you're here. They want you to convince me to give up on my brother" is strongly suggestive of an authoritarian role for ethics consultants, in both of the senses described above. The sister's words imply that the consultant's role is more to *exclude* than to *include* (*process* authoritarianism); more to enforce the substantive moral values the consultant deems to be correct, and see to it that those values drive decision making (*outcome* authoritarianism), than to identify appropriate moral decision makers. All who have done ethics consultation know there is some truth in the charge. Often we are indeed invited into cases because of "difficult" patients, family members, or surrogates, and health care professionals do sometimes see the ethics consultant's role as getting the patient or family member to agree with a proposed course of action (to "come around" or "get on board"). To the extent that we fail to do this, we run the risk of being perceived as ineffectual, or worse.

We should note that an authoritarian approach to ethics consultation (be it to process or outcome) can take another common form quite different from that implied in the case of the Beloved Brother, but equally illegitimate. Sometimes ethics consultants are called in by patients, family members, surrogates, or members of the health care team as sort of "ethics police" or "moral marines." In fact, physicians sometimes oppose ethics consultation precisely because they see it as a means of policing or overseeing their practice or as implying a moral failing on their part.[18] Again, it is understandable why some would hold this view. In popular culture, there is a fairly entrenched view of "ethics" as primarily involving policing or oversight (stemming largely from use of the term in government proceedings). The view that consultants are substantive moral experts whose role is to act as primary decision maker strongly lends itself to the policing or oversight role ("good" ethicists vs. "bad" doctors).

Pure Facilitation Approach

An authoritarian approach, however, is not the only extreme to avoid in ethics consultation. In an effort to neither be nor appear to be authoritarian, consultants run the risk of going to an equally inappropriate extreme that the ASBH report terms *pure facilitation*. According to the report,

> The sole goal of the pure facilitation approach is to forge consensus among involved parties. To illustrate the inadequacies of this approach, imagine that consultants facilitate a consensus between a patient's family and the health care team to override the applicable wishes of the patient as expressed in a valid advance directive. The patient has become unconscious; no other relevant new information has become known. Though the consultants are inclusive and achieve consensus, they do so without clarifying the implications of societal, legal, and institutional values for the case, which have been discussed in detail in the bioethics literature. As the case shows, by merely facilitating consensus, consultants risk forging a consensus that falls outside acceptable boundaries. In this case, the consensus amounts to a violation of the patient's right to self-determination.[19]

Just as the authoritarian approach *usurps* legitimate decision-making authority, the pure facilitation approach *abrogates* it in favor of *merely achieving consensus*. In the case of the Beloved Brother, pure facilitation, if successful, could lead either to withdrawing care, if the family "comes around" to the health care team's view, or to continuing care indefinitely, if the health care team "comes around" to the family's view. We might say that a pure facilitation approach looks for "consensus for the sake of consensus," without independent justification for the course adopted. As the example from the ASBH report illustrates, this can be just as dangerous and illegitimate as an authoritarian approach.

Meeting the Need: Ethics Facilitation

"I know why you're here. They want you to convince me to give up on my brother [she starts to cry], but you don't understand . . . I can never give up on my brother [sobbing] . . . How could you ask me to give up on my brother? How could I live with myself if I gave up on him? I love him so much [her brother comforts her]."[20]

If the argument above is correct, our role in ethics consultation is neither to strong-arm the family or the care team into doing what the other wants, nor to *merely* build a consensus, as if that alone should carry moral and political weight. What *is* our role then? Why *are* we there?

The ASBH report attempts to chart a mean between authoritarian and pure facilitation approaches to ethics consultation with what it terms *ethics facilitation*. I conclude this discussion by looking at the ethics facilitation approach itself, as characterized in the report, and what it would mean for our case. Ultimately, such an approach, I contend, best meets the need for health care ethics consultation as it emerges in our society, while remaining consistent with the fundamental values that drive our liberal constitutional system.

The ASBH report characterizes ethics facilitation in the following way:

We believe an ethics facilitation approach is most appropriate for health care ethics consultation in contemporary society. The ethics facilitation approach is informed by the context in which ethics consultation is done and involves two core features: identifying and analyzing the nature of the value uncertainty and facilitating the building of consensus.

To identify and analyze the nature of the value uncertainty or conflict underlying the consultation, the ethics consultant must:

- gather relevant data (e.g., through discussions with involved parties, examination of medical records or other relevant documents)
- clarify relevant concepts (e.g., confidentiality, privacy, informed consent, best interest)
- clarify related normative issues (e.g., the implications of societal values, law, ethics, and institutional policy for the case)
- help to identify a range of morally acceptable options within the context.

Health care ethics consultants also should help to address the value uncertainty or conflict by facilitating the building of consensus among involved parties (e.g., patients, families, surrogates, health care providers). This requires them to:

- ensure that involved parties have their voices heard
- assist involved individuals in clarifying their own values
- help facilitate the building of morally acceptable shared commitments or understandings within the context.

In contrast to the other approaches, the ethics facilitation approach recognizes the boundaries for morally acceptable solutions normally set by the context in which ethics consultation is done. In contrast to the authoritarian approach, ethics facilitation emphasizes an inclusive consensus-building process. It respects the rights of individuals to live by their own moral values by not misplacing moral decision-making authority or acceding to the personal moral views of the consultant. In contrast to the pure facilitation approach, ethics facilitation recognizes that societal values, law, and institutional policy, often as discussed in the bioethics literature, have implications for a morally acceptable consensus. The ethics facilitation approach is fundamentally consistent with the rights of individuals to live by their own moral values and the fact of pluralism. It, therefore, responds to the need for ethics consultation as it emerges in our society.[21]

As the terminology suggests, "ethics facilitation" involves both "ethics" and "facilitation." Here I emphasize, somewhat artificially, the "ethics" element, since this is what distinguishes the ethics facilitation approach from mere facilitation and, in the context of the clinic, makes illegitimate the authoritarian approaches characterized above.[22] In actual practice, of course, "ethics" and "facilitation" are bound together. In addition, each is of great import, with relative importance in practice being contingent upon the specific details of the case at hand.

In the Beloved Brother case, the motive of the care team was, as the sister suggested, to involve "ethics" so as to convince the sister that it was time to withdraw care, as the team genuinely thought was the right thing to do. However, as we have seen, the role of the ethics consultation team, at least as characterized in the ASBH report, was fundamentally twofold: (1) to identify and analyze the nature of the value conflict or uncertainty at issue in the case by gathering the "facts" of the case, clarifying important concepts and related normative issues, and helping to identify morally acceptable options *within the context*, and (2) to facilitate the building of consensus by ensuring that all parties' voices were heard, assisting those involved to clarify their own values and, if possible, to facilitate the building of morally acceptable shared commitments or understandings *within the context* (the foundation, of course, for a consensus about what should be done). *Within the context*, then, appears to be a key hermeneutic for understanding the ethics facilitation approach.

"Ethics" in clinical ethics consultation is importantly different from academic speculation in ethics. In the comfort of the classroom, one can adopt particular substantive moral views, consider their implications, and argue toward particular conclusions. (This can be done, of course, from any number of substantive moral frameworks—utilitarian, religious, Kantian, virtue ethics, and so forth.) Indeed, in the comfort of the classroom, one may look at the Beloved Brother case and ask "Who is right?" and then make a substantive moral argument incorporating thick values about quality of life or sanctity of life, and so on, to support the care team's view or the sister's view, or another view altogether.

"Ethics" for clinical ethics consultation, however, is profoundly different *even at this theoretical level*, precisely because of its *irreducibly contextual dimensions*. In clinical ethics consultation, issues are framed by certain social and political realities that, even if ignored in the classroom or set to one side for the sake of discussion, must be taken seriously in practical decision making. As the ASBH report underscores, some of these social and political realities, such as fundamental societal values, law, and institutional policy, also carry normative weight and so must inform decision making. Foremost among these is the social and political *fact* that all parties bring to the case certain moral and political rights grounded in our liberal constitutional democratic framework. In clinical ethics consultation, when parties disagree not about the "facts" but about what should be done in the light of those facts (i.e., when people do not share the same values), the focus, given this societal context, should be less on "who *is* right" than on "who *has* the right" (to adapt a famous Dworkinian distinction).[23] Thus, one of the most fundamental ethical questions for actual clinical ethics consultation is often "Who is (or are) the appropriate decision maker(s)?" or, to put it another way, "Whose values should be reflected in decision making?"

In the Beloved Brother case, it would have been best, of course, if the beloved brother could have spoken for himself, because the decision would have been his to make. Why? Recall our discussion at the outset of this chapter about the lack of a privileged substantive moral view in our society, giving to each the right to live his or her life by his or her values. These rights do not evaporate merely because one falls ill and becomes a patient (to paraphrase the ASBH report). Thus, the beloved brother, too, has a moral and political right to live his life by his values, and his values may have implications for medical decision making, as illustrated through the case of the Multitalented Motorcyclist. Interestingly, no matter what any of the rest of us may think about the patient's substantive values—whether or not he *is* "right" in some sense—he still *has* the moral and political *right* to make these decisions; his "having the right" stems from the societal value of autonomy as embedded in our liberal constitutional political structures.

Thus, at least at the theoretical level, a key ethical dimension of the Beloved Brother case would have been much easier to deal with if the beloved brother had been able to speak directly for himself (as *competent* and *well informed*—key concepts that may demand clarification in specific cases), or even indirectly through an applicable advance directive. In the absence of this, "ethics" in the clinical context calls for the identification of an appropriate surrogate. This, of course, raises the question of the surrogate's role in decision making, since one cannot identify an appropriate surrogate without a good grasp of a surrogate's role. Even here, "ethics" in the clinical context differs from "ethics" as academic speculation. In the practical clinical context, our liberal constitutional framework and the autonomy rights it extends to individuals, which may or may not be taken seriously in the comfort of the classroom, both requires that we attempt to identify an appropriate surrogate and helps to *define* the concept itself.[24] In the Beloved Brother case, clarifying the normative concept of *surrogate* proved crucial for reaching a practical resolution of the case, and illustrates well the ethics facilitation approach at work.

In the actual case of the Beloved Brother, the consultation was called by a frustrated nursing staff (as the case description clearly reveals). The first step in carrying out the consultation, then, was to gather the "facts" of the case as accurately as possible and to gather input from involved parties so that we (a physician colleague and I who happened to be on call that month) might have a rounded view of the case. Our initial contact was with the nursing staff, as the head nurse called the consultation. The nurses expressed a great deal of anger toward the sister, saying she was "selfish" and "torturing" her brother. During this initial meeting, one of the nurses broke down and began to cry while relaying her own experience of being intubated and suctioned. She said that every time she suctioned the patient, he grimaced or winced. In discussing the case with the nursing staff, it became clear that they thought the patient's sister loved him but was unable to deal with her own issues of "letting go." They emphasized that they thought it was time for the sister to "give up and move on." The nursing staff also relayed that the patient's brother, though he had lived with the patient for more than thirty years, was usually silent about the situation in deference to his sister. We also learned that the patient was referred to as "Green," an affectionate nickname reflecting his love for gardening and the outdoors.

After discussing the case with the nursing staff, we met briefly with the medical team. Apparently, there was disagreement early on regarding Green's prognosis and the appropriate course of care. At the time of the consultation, however, all doctors involved in Green's care thought the situation was utterly bleak and care should be withdrawn. They revealed that they had continued aggressive therapy only in order to give the sister time to "come around" to accepting that she was going to lose her brother. They echoed the nurses' sentiment that the sister was the "recognized decision maker" in the family and that Green's brother was silent and passive, though he visited Green regularly with his sister.

After a brief discussion with the social worker involved in the case, which reaffirmed what had been relayed to us from the doctors and nurses, we set up a meeting with Green's brother and sister (just the four of us in a private meeting room). The meeting began as described in the case vignette ("I know why you're here"). This was a very powerful opening, and there is, as I have said, some truth in the sister's words. In response, we explained that we thought no one should ask her to give up on her brother, but that our role was to try to understand what was going on and, if possible, to help people come to an agreement about what should be done and why. We explained that we had talked to the doctors and nurses about Green and that we wanted to talk to them, too, so we could understand what they thought was going on. We also emphasized that everybody needed to be thinking about what was best for Green and that we needed to know what the sister and brother thought Green's condition to be. At this point, Green's sister relaxed somewhat and began to talk about his condition. She knew he was very sick, she said, and that the nurses didn't think he would "get better," but one doctor had said "there's a chance he could get better." She then again became upset, saying "and how could I live with myself if I gave up on him, and they want me to give up on him." As she continued to speak, two issues became increasingly evident: her understanding of her brother's prognosis and her view of her own role as his surrogate. Throughout the conversation Green's brother remained silent.

As we discussed with her what she thought the doctor meant by saying there was "a chance" that Green would "get better," it became clear that she thought "chance" meant a significant chance and that "get better" meant almost fully recover, rather than have a modest technical medical improvement. We explained that the doctors had told us Green couldn't get better like that, and we offered to set up a meeting with the doctors so Green's condition could be clarified. The conversation then gradually turned to her role as surrogate decision maker. We told her that no one should be asking her to give up on Green, but what everyone (she and her brother, and all the members of the care team) should try to understand was what Green would have wanted, so that his wishes could be respected. We emphasized that the decision was really *Green's* to make—not the care team's, not ours, not hers, but Green's—and that if she and her brother could help the care team understand what Green would have wanted, that is what should be done. As the discussion continued, it was as if she was beginning to feel a little less burdened, a bit less overwhelmed and more at peace.

We then asked the sister if she had ever talked with Green about this kind of thing, what she thought he would have wanted, or what he might say if he could speak for himself. We asked whether she thought Green would have wanted to go on like this, and at that point a remarkable thing happened. Her brother, who had not said a single word throughout the conversation, suddenly and emphatically blurted out, "Ain't no way Green woulda' wanted this—ain't no way, ain't no way. He hated hospitals and nursing homes and—just ain't no way," and he again fell silent. His sister gave him a look that was at the same time startled, surprised, and a bit apologetic. After a long pause, she seemed to agree, but said she needed time to think things over. She asked us to set up a meeting with the doctors for the next day, at which time she was ready to move forward with comfort measures only. Green died a few days later.

There are several points worth underscoring for the purposes of this chapter. First, this loving sister's words ("I know why you're here. They want you to convince me to give up on my brother") are a challenge to all those involved in ethics consultation to avoid being co-opted into an authoritarian approach that might, albeit subtly, serve to arrogate rather than uphold legitimate decision-making authority. Second, the sister's words also belie a common misunderstanding that surrogates have of their own role in decision making, which itself amounts to a displacement of legitimate decision-making authority. Surrogates often see their role not as trying to choose as the patient would have chosen if able to choose for himself or herself but rather as having the full burden of decision making on their shoulders. In addition to threatening to displace, rather than extend, the legitimate decision-making authority of the patient, this misunderstanding can be emotionally devastating for surrogates. Elsewhere I have described this as follows:

> The crushing burden of end-of-life decision making can be eased somewhat by helping surrogates come to a proper understanding of their role. While no one should ever ask another person to "give up" on his/her loved one, neither should surrogates have to feel that life and death decisions are truly theirs to make. The proper role of surrogates is to help identify the patient's values so that decisions can be made that respect those values. In the actual case upon which this is based, the situation had polarized with the health care team on one side and the patient's sister and brother on the other. The health care team thought it was time to "give up and let go," while the patient's sister said that she would "never give up." The fact that this decision was really the *patient's* was lost in the gravity of the situation. As the patient's sister came to see herself as helping others to understand what her brother would have wanted if he could have made the decision for himself, it was as if a great weight had been lifted from her shoulders . . . A day later, she was ready to withdraw treatment and move forward with comfort measures only. In seeing the decision as, fundamentally, one that should reflect her beloved brother's values, the crushing burden of decision making was lightened. She no longer saw herself as "giving up" on her brother, but rather as respecting the decision he would have made if only able to speak for himself.[25]

Conclusion

Once factual information had been gathered from involved parties in the Beloved Brother case, the normative focus of the ethics facilitation approach on identifying appropriate decision makers and clarifying the proper role for those decision makers helped guide the practical resolution. Indeed, clarifying the concept of *surrogate* in the light of the societal and political context in which decision making must go on in contemporary health care was a key to unburdening the patient's sister and laying the groundwork for the consensus that emerged based on what Green would have wanted. Thus, how the Beloved Brother case might be handled through ethics facilitation stands in stark contrast to how it might be handled through authoritarian and pure facilitation approaches (as characterized and illustrated above). The very features that in part give rise to the need for ethics consultation in the first place, as I argued at the outset of this chapter, inform the ethics facilitation approach at the theoretical level and, at the same time, give practical guidance to how cases might be appropriately resolved. Foremost among these features are the complexities of decision making created by modern health care, the social and political realities of value pluralism, and the rights of individuals to live by their values. The ethics facilitation approach, then, in taking seriously these fundamental contextual features, both is informed by and responds to the need for ethics consultation, as it arises in contemporary health care in our society.

Notes

1. Aulisio, M.P., "Standards for Ethical Decision Making at the End of Life," in *Advance Directives and Surrogate Decision Making in Illinois*, ed. T. May and P. Tudico (Springfield, Ill.: Human Services Press, 1999), pp. 21–34.

2. "Ethics Consultation in U.S. Hospitals," presented by Ellen Fox, M.D., of the National Center for Ethics in Health Care, Department of Veterans Affairs, Washington, D.C., at the Annual Meeting of the American Society for Bioethics and Humanities, Baltimore, October 2002.

3. Cranford, R.E., and Doudera, E.A., "The Emergence of Institutional Ethics Committees," in *Institutional Ethics Committees and Health Care Decision Making*, ed. R.E. Cranford and E.A. Doudera (Ann Arbor, Mich.: Health Administration Press, 1984), pp. 5–21. See also the Joint Commission on Accreditation of Healthcare Organizations (JCAHO), "Patients Rights and Organizational Ethics," in *Comprehensive Accreditation Manual for Hospitals* (Chicago: JCAHO, 1995), p. 66; and JCAHO, *Comprehensive Accreditation Manual for Hospitals* (Chicago: JCAHO, 1997), pp. RI-1–RI-32. For the most recent JCAHO standards and revisions, see the JCAHO web site (www.jcaho.org).

4. Giles Scofield has been the most strident proponent of this view; see his "Here Come the Ethicists!" *Trends in Health Care, Law and Ethics* 8, no. 4 (1993):19–22; and "Ethics Consultation: The Least Dangerous Profession?" *Cambridge Quarterly of Healthcare Ethics* 2, no. 4 (1993):417-26. See also Scofield's "Ethics Consultants, Architects, and Moral Enclosures," *Trends in Health Care, Law and Ethics* 9, no. 4 (1994):7–12; and "Ethics Consultation: The Most Dangerous Profession: A Reply to Critics," *Cambridge Quarterly of Healthcare Ethics* 4, no. 2 (1995):225–28.

5. This hypothetical case is a variation on Lon Fuller's famous case of the Speluncean Explorers, first broached in the *Harvard Law Review* (62 [1949]:616) and often invoked to push the limits of moral theory, be it deontic or consequentialist. For a nice discussion of this case in the context of the criminal law, see chap. 1 of Leo Katz's *Bad Acts and Guilty Minds: Conundrums of the Criminal Law* (Chicago: University of Chicago Press, 1987).

6. See J. Katz's *The Silent World of Doctor and Patient* (New York: Free Press, 1984) for an excellent discussion of the evolution of the legal doctrine of informed consent and related issues.

7. Over the last thirty years, there has been a growing recognition that these rights extend into the domain of health care. While the Patient Self Determination Act of 1991 is perhaps the most explicit recognition of this, countless court cases, requirements of regulatory bodies, and pronouncements of health professional societies have affirmed this as well.

8. I want to thank Thomas May for this simple, but clear, example.

9. Discussions of "competence" or "decision-making capacity" are themselves quite tangled and value-laden. See, for example, Allen E. Buchanan and Dan W. Brock's chapter "Competence and Incompetence," in *Deciding for Others: The Ethics of Surrogate Decision Making* (Cambridge: Cambridge University Press, 1989). For a nice practical guide to assessing competency, see Thomas Grisso and Paul S. Appelbaum's *Assessing Competence to Consent for Treatment: A Guide for Physicians and Other Health Professionals* (Oxford: Oxford University Press, 1998).

10. There is, of course, room for controversy as to whether the patient's valuing of her piano-playing skill is a "moral" or "nonmoral" value (see chapter 3 of Jonathan Dancy's *Moral Reasons* [Cambridge: Blackwell Publishers, 1993] for a brief discussion of the distinction between "moral" and "nonmoral" reasons). Though this is an interesting and important discussion, the distinction is not relevant for our purposes here, as our patient retains the right to live by her values, be they "moral" or "nonmoral" according to some particular conception of value.

11. Nowhere has the current state of moral fragmentation been more powerfully articulated than in H. Tristram Engelhardt's *The Foundations of Bioethics,* 2d ed. (Oxford: Oxford University Press, 1996).

12. Al Jonsen and Stephen Toulmin offer an interesting discussion of this in *The Abuse of Casuistry* (Berkeley: University of California Press, 1988). See also Glenn McGee's "Pragmatic Method and Bioethics," in *Pragmatic Bioethics* (Nashville, Tenn.: Vanderbilt University Press, 1999), pp. 18–29.

13. The Task Force on Standards for Bioethics Consultation endorsed ethics facilitation without taking a position on whether it is better done by individuals, teams, or committees. In Chapter 6 of this volume, Rushton, Youngner, and Skeel argue that a team approach to ethics consultation is optimal.

14. It is important to note that I am deliberately characterizing *extreme* approaches for the purposes of contrast. I am not offering a *description* of particular approaches advocated in the literature.

15. Society for Health and Human Values–Society for Bioethics Consultation: Task Force on Standards for Bioethics Consultation, *Core Competencies for Health Care Ethics Consultation: The Report of the American Society for Bioethics and Humanities* (Glenview, Ill.: American Society for Bioethics and Humanities, 1998), p. 5. (Hereafter cited as ASBH report.)

16. Ibid., pp. 5–6.

17. Ibid., p. 6.

18. I have encountered this concern in my own experience.

19. ASBH report, p. 6.

20. Aulisio, "Standards for Ethical Decision Making," pp. 27–29.

21. ASBH report, pp. 6–7.

22. The facilitation component of ethics facilitation is emphasized more by Arnold and Wilson Silver in Chapter 5.

23. Dworkin, R., *Taking Rights Seriously* (Cambridge: Harvard University Press, 1978).

24. This is true in all states, but it is especially pronounced in states (e.g., Illinois and Ohio) that have laws specifying a hierarchy of surrogacy.

25. Aulisio, "Standards for Ethical Decision Making," p. 30.

2

Can Ethics Consultation Be Saved?

Ethics Consultation and Moral Consensus in a Democratic Society

JONATHAN MORENO, PH.D.

"These decisions [concerning ethical problems] must be made in a pluralistic society in which individuals have the right, based on the value of autonomy, to pursue their own conception of the good."[1] With these words, *Core Competencies for Health Care Ethics Consultation,* the report of the ASBH, declares itself a child of the Enlightenment. The spirit of this passage should come as no surprise to bioethics watchers. As I have argued elsewhere, the bioethics movement is characterized by several themes familiar to American philosophizing. These themes include not only the more obvious one of personal autonomy that the Founders derived from John Locke, but also the more subtle and equally important bioethical assumption that moral experience can help us define our values and refine our ethical choices. Little noticed at the heart of bioethics is a wildly successful merger of Continental liberalism with early twentieth-century American pragmatism, of democratic individualism with an experimental theory of moral knowledge. If I am right, this conjunction will drive any adequate account of ethics consultation in a liberal society.

In such an account, not only liberalism but also the form that a liberal solution to social conflict assumes will be reflected. Thus, through several papers and a book, *Deciding Together,*[2] I developed a theory of the role of ethics committees in a liberal democratic society. In that theory, ethics committees are viewed as instruments for the construction of moral consensus in modern bureaucratic medical institutions that routinely deal with the gravest ethical issues, under conditions that combine powerful technology with residual uncertainty. In this chapter I focus specifically on ethics consultation. How does ethics consultation enable individuals to "pursue their own conception of the good"? What are the hazards along the way, and how can ethics consultation (and Enlightenment moral philosophy itself) avoid moral relativism and spiritual bankruptcy? My approach is fallibilist: perfection in this area cannot be achieved, and any specific moral arrangement is subject to revision in the light of new information, novel arguments, or unintended consequences. Ethics consultation should be guided by certain procedural values that are widely embraced, at least in Western culture Among these values are a nonviolent approach to resolving moral controversies, respect for differences of opinion, and a willingness to entertain opposing points of view.

The approach taken in this chapter, and that of the Task Force on Standards for Bioethics Consultation itself, is of course not the only analytical framework from which to assess the practice of ethics consultation. Specific ethical criteria may also be applied to such an assessment. For example, Edmund Pellegrino has forcefully argued that the patient's good rather than consensus should remain in the forefront of ethics consultation.[3] In a pluralistic society, what should count as appropriate ethical criteria is often precisely what is at issue. The same may be said about what counts as the good of the patient. Therefore, I do not view my project as incompatible with efforts to assess ethics consultation according to particular ethical criteria.

Ethics Consultation and the Pursuit of the Good

Classical liberalism aims to construct a public space that is neutral in its conception of the good life, so individuals can pursue their preferences. An ethics consultation practice that would most obviously conflict with the liberal agenda would be that which advanced a certain single-minded conception of the good life. Consider, for example, the view that every moment of life is of infinite value and therefore that life must be preserved at all costs. Or consider the view that a utilitarian calculus must be applied to evaluate the worth of extending a life that deviates from some standard of normalcy. Held by an ethics consultant, a vitalist philosophy that any life is of inestimable good clearly has implications for his or her practice, as does a utilitarian view that the value of life is always subject to estimation.

A conflict between what I have characterized as the liberal agenda for ethics consultation and a single-minded view of the good life could occur either consciously and deliberately or in an unconscious and non-self-critical manner. At its extreme, the deliberate rejection of moral pluralism calls to mind pulpit-pounding jeremiads, but it can also manifest in a more subtle and intellectually challenging way. On a recent trip to Israel I was pressed hard by some orthodox Jews on what they saw as the foundationless nature of America's secular medical morality. I responded that in the American context, if there is no successful pluralistic morality there can be no morality, and the latter is not an acceptable alternative. Impressed if not persuaded, my interlocutors nevertheless reminded me that there can be no substitute for arguing from a rich body of received and internally coherent law. If in our pluralistic society there is a secret longing for such a framework, we are doomed to disappointment.

In my conversation in Israel I did not pursue the point that even within a certain faith tradition, we find differences of opinion on the interpretation of shared values. For many believers, these differences play an important role in animating the adventure that is religious faith. Even commitment to a single body of religious law is no guarantee of wholesale agreement, but disagreements that are matters of interpretation are of a different logical order than disagreements that stem from differing value systems. In the former circumstance, there is nothing inappropriate or misleading in members of the clergy taking the role of de facto ethics consultant; that is, in fact, precisely what they are meant to do. Besides subscription to the same coherent body of principles, this kind of social arrangement also requires acceptance of a certain structure of authority for settling areas of potentially disputed interpretation. All in all, the very idea of an ethics consultant seems somehow out of place or at least redundant in a faith community, with its system of relatively well-defined and internally consistent values that are widely accepted. This conclusion returns us to the intuition that the ethics consultation role—at least, in the way it has been defined in the United States—only makes sense in a context of liberal pluralistic individualism.

To see that ethics consultation as commonly conceived is mainly at home in an American-style setting, consider what skills are demanded of its practitioners. Not only cognitive skills, such as familiarity with ethical principles, are demanded of the ethics consultant, but also interpersonal skills, such as an ability to help people find common ground on which to build acceptable solutions to controversies. To be sure, the ethics consultant does generally appear to be *an authority,* derived from her or his social status as a highly trained and titled professional. However, to appeal to an old philosophical distinction, this is a far cry from being "in authority" (i.e., one who has the social standing to command a solution). Rather, the ethics consultant must finally rely on an originality and creativity not ordinarily demanded of theocrats.

Although liberalism could not tolerate a theocracy, it does of course permit and even encourage private associations of individuals who share a certain conception of the good. Though private and voluntary associations, the institutions that result may also be engaged in public service. A relevant example is health care institutions that declare themselves to be in allegiance with certain faith traditions. These entities not only may self-identify as, say, Catholic or

Jewish, they may also be affiliated with religious organizations in the same organized faith community, such as a specific archdiocese or social service group. At the same time they are often open for business to all comers, without requiring that their clients identify themselves with that faith tradition.

Unlike voluntary associations embedded within a larger society that subscribes to the same system of moral values and to a system of interpretive authorities, these faith-centered institutions are routinely encountered by individuals who may not identify with or even be cognizant of their moral commitments. In at least some instances, institutional values will not permit the provision of services on demand. Familiar examples are certain reproductive services in a Roman Catholic institution (e.g., abortion and in vitro fertilization) and certain end-of-life procedures in a Jewish hospital (e.g., forgoing life-sustaining treatment). In the former example the controversial services are "elective" and therefore their provision is not strictly obligatory, but they may be otherwise unavailable in a surrounding community that is not wholly or even predominantly Catholic. In the latter example, dying patients who do not subscribe to orthodox views of life-prolongation cannot easily be transferred to another facility.

A nice question virtually absent from bioethical discussion is how ethics consultants should operate in sectarian hospitals embedded within a secular society, and who those consultants should be. Are they advocates for the values of the hospital? Should they represent those values to the community of actual and potential patients? Are they to find ways to accommodate their institutional policies to secular interests?

Provisionally, it appears that religiously identified institutions that seek to do business in a pluralistic society should make some accommodation to their environment. Though they need not be forced to abandon deeply held principles that provide their distinct identity, sectarian institutions do enjoy the benefits of the society in which they exist, and members of the community being served are stakeholders with legitimate interests in the treatment options available to them. At the very least, it seems harsh that patients who find themselves with no practical alternative but admission to a hospital affiliated with a faith community that is not their own (as is often the case) must therefore be wholly deprived of the opportunity to select treatment in accord with their own values. In such circumstances ethics consultants may have an important role as mediators between the sectarian institution and the patient community that is representative of the secular society in which the institution functions.

These forms of deliberate rejection of the liberal agenda entail substantive views of the good life. By contrast, one may think of oneself as a proper member of a liberal democratic society and yet suffer from an unconscious failure to embrace pluralism—wedded to one's own point of view while thinking oneself to be open-minded. In many social roles, unreflective commitment to a particular standpoint is acceptable if not laudable. But in ethics consultation this very human tendency will not do at all, not in a society founded on Enlightenment liberalism.

Morality and Democracy

For a certain classical tradition of philosophy, the conjunction of morality and democracy is a frank self-contradiction. One of the great intellectual dramas of Western culture is the confrontation between the individual with actual insight into the good and the blind mob. It is a pattern played out time and again: Moses, Socrates, Jesus, Joan of Arc, Gandhi, and Martin Luther King are among the protagonists. In particular, Socrates in his trial and in the circumstances of his death embodied this tragic tale at the heart of Western epistemology, one that Plato transformed into a metaphysic and Augustine into a theology. It is no accident that the institutions shaped by Plato and Augustine—the academy and the church—are both characterized by authority and hierarchy rather than popular preference.

There was, of course, another element in classical anthropology, one that was implicit and often suppressed. This other element celebrated the potential for at least some individuals to transcend their perceptual limitations and appreciate that which is true and good—to "see the light" as did Moses on Mt. Sinai and Plato's philosopher-kings. This divine spark could hardly be denied (on pain of self-contradiction), although few could realistically hope to share in it. Nonetheless, there was a basis here for the elevation of all who shared in being human. It is this aspect of classical philosophy, the suppressed but essential humanism, that inspired the *philosophes* and gave the Enlightenment an entering wedge to liberal individualism.

Many of the intellectuals who were indebted to the rediscovery of the possibility of human transcendence nonetheless retained a certain reserve about the promise of liberalism. Shakespeare has Hamlet say, "What a piece of work is man! How noble in reason!" while the audience presumably shares the irony that few actual human beings achieve the exalted status for which their nature gives them potential. Kant builds his philosophical masterpiece on the human capacity to self-legislate the moral law, otherwise known as autonomy, but he doesn't suggest that autonomy is a typical or even common human condition. Reading between the lines of his moral philosophy one has quite the opposite impression.

The notion that self-determination can (and should) characterize human society is the distinctive contribution of the English philosophers. Here we find an equivocal and critical transition from autonomy as Kant understood it to self-determination as the political philosophers understood it. Adam Smith's "invisible hand" thesis in political economy helps justify the equivocation, for according to Smith there is harmony between the self-determined/self-interested behavior of individuals and the laws of the economic universe within which they interact. If each pursues his or her own good, matters tend to work out: supply and demand balance, prices fall and quality rises, and value distributes itself evenly throughout the marketplace.

To be sure, the English empiricists were not relativists about the good, Jeremy Bentham's utilitarian calculus being perhaps the most famous counter-example to such a notion. And though Smith is commonly cited as the god-father of the free market, *The Wealth of Nations* also deplores a society in which only private interests rule in the public realm. But in matters concerning social organization, the empiricists were mainly political rather than moral philosophers, and in that context the dominant notion was that of a social compact of discrete individuals each with her or his own moral status and deserving of respect and a suitable zone of privacy.

To put my view simply, in our philosophical tradition autonomy is a moral notion but self-determination is a political one. To be autonomous is to be a self-legislator of the moral law, to be self-determining is to be able to act on one's authentic preferences. In this sense, liberal democrats from Locke to the American Founders had not autonomy but self-determination in mind as the key element in the liberal polity. To be sure, this story is a complicated one, because the Jeffersonian-Lockean appeal to "self-evidence" of human equality does suggest a transcendent moral order, but a very minimal one that specifies little beyond "life, liberty, and the pursuit of happiness."

More detailed conceptions of the moral order as sketched by the Founders in the Declaration of Independence are of course possible, but not prescribed. Associations of members of the polity may include those based on common moral standpoints; herein lies the critical role of moral consensus (usually of a passive and implicit variety rather than active and self-conscious as in much social contract theory). But surely it would be too much to insist that all those common moral standpoints be expressive of the moral law. Though such would be an outcome devoutly to be wished, it is not one on which a liberal democracy can insist, for then it comes to look very much like Plato's aristocracy.

I belabor this point about the transition from Kantian autonomy to empiricist self-determination because without an appreciation of this move it is easy to misunderstand the role of bioethicists when, like ethics consultants, they are social actors. Confusion on this point can lead to a multitude of other errors, such as confusing ethics consultants with "moralists," those whose purpose is to persuade concerning a particular moral standpoint, using any rhetorical means necessary. To be sure, there are moral constraints on ethics consultants, but they are rooted in the political values of classical liberalism, not the perceived duties of persons called to action.

Hazards along the Way

In a formal sense, the values to which ethics consultation in a liberal society should aspire are those that are essential to democratic procedures when moral controversy arises. These values include a nonauthoritarian attitude toward moral questions, a respectful and nonviolent attitude toward disagreement, and a willingness to consider all relevant points of view. This is the burden of my argument so far, one that squares with what the ASBH report calls the "ethics facilitation" approach. Among the elements of this approach are "an inclusive consensus-building process," "not misplacing moral decision-making authority or acceding to the personal moral views of the consultant," and recognizing that "societal values, law, and institutional policy . . . have implications for a morally acceptable consensus." On the whole, ethics facilitation is said to be "fundamentally consistent with the rights of individuals to live by their own moral values and the fact of pluralism."[4]

I have also urged that the form ethics consultation has taken in our liberal society is rooted in political values. In the report's general statement of the goal of health care ethics consultation, a critical phrase is the "resolution of ethical issues," specified as the "resolution of conflicts."[5] Conflict resolution is not a chapter in any substantive moral philosophy, but it is a method for managing deep differences without recourse to violence. What defines the consultative situation as involving ethics is not that it is resolved by reference to a particular moral theory (this would be what the report calls an "authoritarian approach") but that the controversial subject matter concerns conflicting *moral* values. At the other extreme, the absence of *any* side constraints (such as certain deep-seated moral precepts) in the pursuit of conflict resolution is characterized as "pure facilitation," which is also rejected in the report. Again, the ethics consultation process is not a value-neutral one, but its values are mainly procedural, a view that emerges directly from classical liberalism.

A notorious difficulty with procedural values is that while in themselves they may be unobjectionable and even trivial (how can anyone disagree with considering all relevant points of view?), they can in their very blandness conceal certain presuppositions that have very substantive consequences. One problem along these lines is that the participants must be self-critical enough to appreciate when they have been co-opted, when they have lost their self-critical faculty, and thus not only are unable to weigh arguments in a disinterested manner but are even unaware of their bias. Similarly, the way that procedures are institutionalized can help ensure that the status quo, which may be patently unjust, is largely impervious to fundamental change.

These criticisms of a system based on procedural values that are unobjectionable on their face are reminiscent of the New Left critiques of the 1960s, which were themselves based on Old Left analyses of bourgeois liberalism by Frankfurt School philosophers.[6] For these thinkers, Nazism was the logical outcome of the Enlightenment. Largely forgotten in the post–Berlin Wall era, the New Leftists updated the critique of Enlightenment liberal values. They argued that procedurally democratic exercises in which everyone could have a say, including the CIA and Army recruiters, effectively blocked change of a racist and economically oppressive society. Supposedly open and free events were effectively co-opted by and served the purposes of the surrounding System (and especially the ruling elites), which rolled right on while the masses suffered and the speechifying continued. The radicals used this analysis as the excuse to prevent "free speech" on campus, much to the dismay of their liberal professors, because the means of protest that were socially acceptable boiled down to no efficacious protest at all.

The New Left account was less subtle but essentially the same as the "critical theory" social analysis of neo-Marxists. Marx himself observed that bourgeois capitalism has the remarkable capacity to transform the world into its own image. Marx turned out to be more right than even he could have known. Consider, for example, the antiestablishment hippie movement, which generated a huge market in the arts and fashion that is still producing capital, paradigmatically embodied in the late 1960s automobile sales pitch delivered by a provocatively dressed model posing seductively on the hood of a new car:

"Join the Dodge Rebellion!" Sex and revolution were effectively turned toward the sale of polluting and unsafe vehicles.

In this spirit, it is noteworthy that for-profit hospitals and entrepreneurial genetic research companies have embraced ethics committees, ethics consultation services, and ethics advisory boards. Were critical theorists to write about the institutionalization of bioethics (which none has done, so far as I know), they could truly have a field day. So long as ethics consultants agree to "play nice" according to the civilized procedural values endorsed by liberalism, not only are they no danger to corporate interests but, these critics would argue, they actually serve those interests by providing ethical cover. Moreover, by being touted and largely recognized within an institution as the font of ethical wisdom, the ethics consultant with sound interpersonal skills and a modicum of intellectual capacity can be a formidable power center. Thus is his or her co-optation complete.

These kinds of accusations have been thrown at ethics consultation for years, of course, and they don't require any reference to neo-Marxist philosophy. Recall the *New Republic* article about ethics consultation by a journalist apparently in search of an intellectual scandal.[7] The critique I am sketching is not a journalistic cheap shot, however. It follows from a comprehensive, substantive world view, as did the complaints about American bioethics lodged by my rabbinical interlocutors. This kind of critique of classical liberalism—that its procedural solution to controversy lacks moral foundation and therefore opens it to evil, recognized or not—goes well beyond an attack on ethics consultation to the core of the liberal world view itself.

Avoiding Moral Relativism and Spiritual Bankruptcy

As I have urged in some of my other writings, I don't believe that bioethics in general, and ethics consultation in particular, has worked hard enough at understanding and responding to this kind of critique. No field that is considered to be a moral resource for problems of actual decision making with potentially grave consequences can spend too much time worrying about its own interests and prejudices. What, then, is a constructive attitude that can be adopted toward what might appear to be a devastating critique? The ASBH report presents an occasion for ethics consultants to focus with renewed intellectual honesty on the conditions that can enable their practice to flourish as well as fatefully undermine it.

First, persons engaged in ethics consultation should continue to take their own potentially morally compromised positions seriously. They should exercise a keen awareness of their economically and socially advantaged position and of the source of their power. They may not be able to assume, as the task force apparently does, that they can effectively facilitate consensus even when they have power over the outcome. For, as Edmund Howe observes, "This presupposition flies in the face of conventional wisdom from other contexts," such as psychotherapy and research.[8] Further, ethics consultants should not delude themselves, or those who have a stake in their activities (especially patients and their families), that institutional authorities are disinterested observers of the work of ethics consultation. In his discussion of organizational ethics, Pellegrino is especially critical of the report for failing to take sufficient note of the conflicts of interest to which ethics consultants may be subject due to their employment by the hospital.[9] An example might be that of a board-level decision to eliminate a socially valuable but loss-leading service: can an ethics consultant express a candid public view about such a policy? To some extent the answer to this question will vary with local circumstances. On the whole, however, it would appear that ethics consultants need to appreciate that the role they play will be welcome so long as it appears to correspond to the long-term interests of the system in which they function. Even then, short-term concerns will prevail in some instances, and ethics consultants can expect either to be shown the door or, more likely, simply to be quietly undermined and ignored.

Second, those who engage in ethics consultation would be wise to remind one another of the precarious intellectual situation that accompanies what is in effect a secular priesthood. They should be their own harshest critics and hold their practice to exacting standards. Hence, Judith Wilson Ross worries that the standards may consist of nothing more than what ethics consultants already know about what they do.[10] They should be concerned that those who seek their counsel, whether patients and families or other professionals, appreciate the complexity of the consultant's role and the fact of her or his human limitations. Of course, this kind of self-criticism can too easily degenerate into an empty ritual or an orgy of mutual denunciation. One way to avoid this problem while meeting the goals I advocate is to expand the study of the ethics consultant's role in the health care organization. Ethics consultants could benefit from an infusion of social science in their ongoing self-examination. What is it to be an ethics "witness" in a complex, modern institution, and how does that role condition the ways in which the social environment responds to the ethics consultant's activities?[11] In general, an understanding of the health care institution as a social system could enhance the effectiveness of the ethics consultant's interventions.[12]

Third, while they pursue these continuing remedies, ethics consultants can take heart—but not too much—from another credo of the twentieth century. For just as the Marxists and their descendants were warning about the materially based limits of moral perception, so the existentialists were touting the necessity of moral choice. "Not to choose is to choose" is a compelling slogan, one that captures the inevitability of personal responsibility for one's actions and their consequent moral nature. Although many of the outstanding existential figures were often aligned with Marxists on political questions, their position on the implicitly moral character of all choice was a two-edged sword for other leftists. On the one hand it was consistent with the message that acquiescence to an oppressive status quo was tantamount to endorsing it. On the other hand it also helped counter the moral paralysis that could accompany a thoroughgoing self-criticism, of the kind I sketched above.

The trouble is that just as existentialist writers embraced the implicit morality of all human action, they also rejected the rationalist epistemology they inherited, especially the transcendental philosophy of Kant. Having jettisoned the foundations of morality according to this, the dominant philosophical system of their culture, they could see no alternative to a moral fatalism. The search for moral foundations is noble but illusory, in this view. For the existentialists this position implied not moral relativism but rather that morality is irrational. For unlike relativists, with whom they have often been confused, existentialists contend that one had better be damned careful what moral choices one makes because they define what one is, and (as the Second World War confirmed) there is simply nothing more important than that.

Clearly, modern bioethicists are neither moral relativists nor existentialists, or at least they don't generally fancy themselves as such. Though they are deeply interested in cultural differences and believe that reference to them may be critical, bioethicists generally resist the notion that in the final analysis all morality is context-dependent. Existentialism also gets no traction in bioethics, because of the presumption in the field that there are better and worse reasons for moral choice and there is such a thing as moral expertise. While they may reject foundational*ism*, perhaps following the explications of Richard Rorty,[13] bioethicists clearly do subscribe to an idea of multiple, practical (and not necessarily changeless) *foundations*, especially where public policy is concerned.

As descendants of Enlightenment liberalism, ethics consultants rely on foundations that are, once again, mainly process values. Those who reject these values (nonviolent solutions to moral controversies, open-mindedness, and so forth) need to come up with better ones. Because bioethicists and ethics consultants reject the absurdity of morality à la existentialism just as they reject the moral paralysis that can follow a self-denouncing neo-Marxism, they are obliged to embrace some guiding principles. Invocations of existential absurdity or class-consciousness are not likely to seem helpful in the patient-management conference.

Talk of foundations is commonly associated with absolutism. But Enlightenment liberals also believe that absolutisms are equally unhelpful in contexts of moral choice that are often tragic, and it is important that much of liberal thought has been engaged in finding ways to steer between rigidity and the insecurity that comes with shifting foundations. The classical emphasis on procedural rather than substantive values is one example of this effort, as are more recent attempts to spell out the specification of moral principles, and the popular philosophical notion of reflective equilibrium. The paradigmatic American gloss on liberal thought, the naturalistic empiricism of the so-called pragmatists, views moral experience as an iterative process in which values guide practice and consequences shape our understanding of values.[14] These examples could be multiplied.

Conclusion

Can ethics consultation be saved from its obvious shortcomings? The approach I take rules out salvation in favor of improvement. Some obvious measures are consistent with the procedural values and the experimental perspective I have described. Ethics consultants must advance a nonviolent, reasoned approach and must defend it as a *sine qua non*. They should ensure that all voices with a purchase on the case have been heard. They should encourage the protagonists to actively consider other points of view, including articulating the reasons they reject them. And they should practice what they preach by accepting and even soliciting feedback on their interventions. Ethics consultants who work as solo practitioners should periodically invite colleagues to audit and critique their work.

The ASBH task force's conception of ethics consultation in a liberal society is aspirational, as evidenced by the report's emphasis on ethics consultants' "self-awareness regarding how their views affect consultation." There is as much art as science in ethics consultation. Perfection is well beyond even our imaginative grasp. Therefore continual improvement (the marks of which are themselves sure to engender controversy) is the most a practice such as ethics consultation can offer. But when matters are as grave as those that often fall within the ambit of ethics consultation, a self-critical process is also the least a pluralistic society should expect.

Notes

1. Society for Health and Human Values–Society for Bioethics Consultation: Task Force on Standards for Bioethics Consultation, *Core Competencies for Health Care Ethics Consultation: The Report of the American Society for Bioethics and Humanities* (Glenview, Ill.: American Society for Bioethics and Humanities), 1998, p. 5.

2. Moreno, J.D., *Deciding Together: Bioethics and Moral Consensus* (New York: Oxford University Press, 1995).

3. Pellegrino, E., "Clinical Ethics Consultations: Some Reflections on the Report of the SHHV-SBC," *Journal of Clinical Ethics* 10, no. 1 (1999):5–12.

4. ASBH report, p. 7.

5. Ibid., p. 8.

6. Horkheimer, M., and Adorno, T.W., *Dialectic of Enlightenment,* trans. J. Cumming (New York: Continuum International Publishing Group, 1976).

7. Shalit, R., "When We Were Philosopher-Kings," *New Republic,* 28 April 1997.

8. Howe, E.G., "Ethics Consultants: Could They Do Better?" *Journal of Clinical Ethics* 10, no. 1 (1999):13–25, see p. 14.

9. Pellegrino, "Clinical Ethics Consultations," p. 11.

10. Ross, J.W., "The Task Force Report: Comprehensible Forest or Unknown Beetles?" *Journal of Clinical Ethics* 10, no. 1 (1999):28–29.

11. Moreno, *Deciding Together,* pp. 140–41.

12. Gallagher, E.B., Schlomann, P., Sloan, R.S., Mesman, J., Brown, J.B., and Cholewinska, A., "To Enrich Bioethics, Add One Part Social to One Part Clinical," in *Bioethics and Society,* ed. R. DeVries and J. Subedi (Upper Saddle River, N.J.: Prentice Hall, 1998).

13. Rorty, R., *Philosophy and the Mirror of Nature* (Princeton: Princeton University Press, 1980).

14. Moreno, J.D., "Bioethics Is a Naturalism," in *Pragmatism and Bioethics,* ed. G. McGee (Nashville, Tenn.: Vanderbilt University Press, 1999).

3

Character and Ethics Consultation

Even the Ethicists Don't Agree

FRANÇOISE BAYLIS, PH.D., HOWARD BRODY, M.D., PH.D.,
MARK P. AULISIO, PH.D., DAN W. BROCK, PH.D., AND
WILLIAM WINSLADE, J.D., PH.D.

All members of the Task Force on Standards for Bioethics Consultation agreed that, in addition to the core competencies, good character is important for optimal ethics consultation. The rationale for this belief, and opinions about the specific relationship between character and ethics consultation, depend on a number of issues on which task force members were divided. This disagreement stemmed, at least in part, from the close connection between character and conceptions of "the good." When people disagree about conceptions of the good, they are also likely to hold divergent conceptions of character.

In task force discussions of character, controversy emerged over whether

- character is a set of observable behaviors, an internalized inclination to behave in a certain way, or a more fundamental constituent of persons
- certain traits of character are necessary for, or incidental to, the acquisition of certain kinds of skills or knowledge that may be important for various activities
- behavior can be compartmentalized so that bad behavior in one domain does not mean that it will be exhibited in other domains
- the better measure of character involves day-to-day activities or extreme tests such as those times when one must take a stand at considerable personal risk
- evaluations of bioethics consultation or consultants need to focus on more than behavior
- character traits can be correctly defined.[1]

As this passage clearly shows, discussions of "character" within the task force were highly contentious. Though all agreed that "good character" or "virtue" is important for "optimal" ethics consultation, this is where the agreement stopped. In some ways, this fragmentation is not surprising as it merely reflects a broader societal divide across the same issues. There is a sense in which everyone agrees that good character is important and desirable, not just for ethics consultants or some select few, of course, but for all persons. There is another sense, however, in which, as a society, we are very uncomfortable talking about character. We have seen this time and again in recent political events. We as a society disagreed about "good" and "bad" character, "public" and "private" behavior, and their relevance for "going about the business of the people," as a great drama was played out on a very public stage by Bill Clinton, Ken Starr, and others. Character later became an issue in the subsequent presidential election as one side pledged to "restore honor and decency to the office" and the other pledged to take up the noble task of "fighting for those without a voice," while both dredged up the other's transgressions and moral failings.

Given the broader societal disagreement about character, then, it is not surprising that this disagreement was reflected, on a smaller scale, in task force discussions about the importance of character for health care ethics consultation. But one might hope that at least the "ethicists"—the very people to whom we sometimes turn to help sort through moral issues—could come to some agreement about the importance of character for something as circumscribed as ethics consultation. Unfortunately or not, depending on your point of view, this was not the case. This chapter, then, is appropriately divided into two parts. In the first part, Françoise Baylis and Howard Brody argue that character is centrally important to the role ethics consultants should play in health care settings. They go so far as to suggest that character or virtue is more central to the ethics consultant's role than to the roles played by health professionals. They do not suggest, and indeed they explicitly reject, the view that ethics consultants are more virtuous than others in health care. In the second part, Mark Aulisio, Dan Brock, and William Winslade take a very different tack. After pointing out some of the vexed problems inherent in discussions of "character" or "virtue," such as profound definitional issues, they argue that expanding the role of ethics consultants to include being role models or exemplars of virtue, as do Baylis and Brody, begs for an answer to the questions "Whose virtue? Which character?"—and in so doing threatens to undermine the role for ethics consultation laid out in the ASBH report itself.

The Importance of Character for Ethics Consultants
FRANÇOISE BAYLIS AND HOWARD BRODY

The current bioethics literature presents two predominant theoretical approaches to health care ethics consultation: ethics consultation as an exercise in adjudicating conflicting rights claims within society, and ethics consultation as an exercise in values clarification. Those of us who work as health care ethics consultants, however, know that neither of these theoretical models fully captures the nature and complexity of practice. Ethics consultation is not simply about conflict resolution and the parsing of rights, nor does it simply require the facilitation of decision makers. Were this all that it involved, then arguments about the importance of character for health care ethics consultation would be neither credible nor persuasive. In our view, ethics consultation is a practice that properly attends to claims and dilemmas of duty, and, precisely because of this, we maintain that certain traits of character or specific virtues are central to the role of the ethics consultant.

A model of health care ethics consultation grounded in duty instead of rights was recently outlined by Benjamin Freedman. He described ethics consultation as a sort of communal call to duty. In his words, "An ethical consultation is best understood as an effort on the part of those caring for a patient to discover what their obligations to the patient require and how these obligations can best be satisfied."[2] Some important conclusions follow from this model. First, according to Freedman, "the duty perspective insists that the right thing be done, and done in the right way, by or with the involvement of the right person."[3] If it is important that the right person does what duty requires, and does it in the right way, then clearly character and virtue are central concerns of the process. It is not enough merely to discern by abstract reason what ought to be done. The involved parties are not being asked merely to determine, as onlookers, what would be the right thing to do in a particular situation; they are being asked instead to rise to the occasion as actors or participants.

Second, with Freedman's model, the health care ethics consultant is "no less the object of duties than those others with whom he consults."[4] That is, the consultant himself is among the involved parties being asked to do his duty. His personal character is on the line along with the characters of all the other parties. In our view, "whether" and "how" the ethics consultant does his duty "is ultimately a function of who he is, how he perceives and confronts moral situations of uncertainty and conflict, and what he is committed to."[5]

Third, something that may be less obvious with the duty-centered view of ethics consultation, is the importance of a biographical perspective on what ethics requires of us. To be a virtuous person is not merely to act, more often than not, in the morally correct way. Rather, it is to devote one's lifetime to becoming a certain sort of person—a person who accurately and creatively discerns what virtue requires in each new situation, and proceeds accordingly, seamlessly and effortlessly. The virtuous person never rests on past accomplishments but always strives to do better, in part because as one's discernment improves with experience, one becomes more adept at spotting even minor lapses. On this view, developing one's character is integral to the practice of health care ethics consultation.

The Task Force on Standards for Bioethics Consultation considered character sufficiently relevant to list examples of character traits associated with successful ethics consultations: (1) tolerance, patience, and compassion, (2) honesty, forthrightness, and self-knowledge, (3) courage, (4) prudence and humility, and (5) integrity.[6] For obvious reasons these traits were not ranked. But, in our view, if there are "cardinal" virtues of ethics consultation, they may well be courage and integrity.

To put it somewhat crudely, most of us find it relatively easy to provide an independent moral voice when we are not at risk of losing anything in the process. But when calling into question the moral acceptability of certain practices, decisions, institutional structures, or policies may have serious personal and professional consequences, the ethics consultant may find it much harder to heed the call of moral duty. For example, there can be considerable economic pressure on ethics consultants: "Working at the intersection between conflicting claims of patients, staff, and administration, bioethicists must often find themselves under pressure to compromise their ideals, to 'get along by going along.' Practically by definition, bioethics treats of issues on which reasonable persons disagree. Sometimes, one such reasonable person will be paying the salary of the other."[7] Judith Andre also writes about the threat of job loss for ethics consultants who are employed by those to whom they offer counsel. She adds that while economic pressures are probably diffused for ethics committee members (unlike for persons employed primarily as ethicists), some committee members (e.g., nurses and allied health professionals) may nonetheless feel vulnerable to retaliation.[8]

More generally, it is often the nature of ethics consultation that the persons providing the consultation service wield less power than those whose practices may be under review or whose practices may have to be altered as a result of the consultation. And so, even in the absence of any explicit threat to job security, the ethics consultant may naturally shrink from upsetting those on whom she depends for information (and often good will) in order to do her job well. But as one of us has argued elsewhere, "An effective health care ethics consultant . . . is not a compliant colleague. S/he needs courage to take a stand in the face of serious wrong, and courage to persevere in the face of seemingly constant 'setbacks, weariness, difficulties and dangers.' Courage inclines the ethics consultant away from a self-centered concern for security."[9]

A good health care ethics consultant is also a person of integrity; a person with the courage of her convictions who will carry out the process of ethics consultation in an even-handed, thoughtful, and effective way, withstanding "bribes and threats, authoritative demands, reproach and accusations of unreasonableness . . . social incredulity, ostracism, [and] contempt."[10] In the face of coercion or temptation, she will not give in or accede to views she does not hold, she will not abandon or compromise the views she does hold, nor will she retreat to silence in an attempt to placate others.[11] Rather, she will speak and act in a manner consistent with her deeply held and cherished beliefs and values.[12] At the same time, because integrity is a social as well as a personal virtue, and because she has taken on special commitments as an ethics consultant, she will, in addition to *standing by* her principles and values, *stand for* principles and values that in her best judgment must be defended "because they concern how *we,* as beings interested in living justly and well, can do so."[13]

So far we have shown that one cannot ignore issues of character and virtue when discussing health care ethics consultation. One might object, however, that we have failed to show that good character is *central* to ethics consultation. All persons who work in health care institutions, and who undertake responsibility for the care of sick and vulnerable human beings, ought to be persons of good character; this hardly demonstrates any difference between the ethics consultant and any other member of staff. Isn't it still true that a person of indifferent moral character, possessed of excellent reasoning skills and well versed in the relevant bioethics literature, could accurately decide what duty requires in any given case? Maybe that person would stumble somewhat in doing what duty required in exactly the right way or in involving all of the right people; but aren't those less important niceties within the process as a whole?

One way to reply to this objection, and at the same time to clarify a critically important question of character, is to make the claim even stronger by insisting that *good character overall, not merely good character in one's professional role,* is required for proper health care ethics consulting. A question that the task force addressed at some length in its internal deliberations was: could a good ethics consultant cheat on his income tax?[14] At first glance, the safest answer seems to be that cheating (or not) on one's income tax is a "private" matter, distinct from one's work in a health care institution. One can imagine, for example, an income tax cheat who nevertheless performs in exemplary fashion as a health care provider, even to the point of being scrupulously honest in all dealings and documentation within the health care institution. Thus it seems that tax cheating can be completely compartmentalized and separated from one's professional role.

But our position on the centrality of character for health care ethics consultation requires that we not take this easy way out. In our view, ethics consultants should not cheat on their income tax, and they should not do so in part *because of* what is required to be a good ethics consultant (in addition to other ethical, legal, and social reasons against such cheating). To be a person of integrity is, in part, to be a whole, integrated self—a person living a cohesive life with coherence between desires, evaluations, commitments, and actions. On this view of integrity, we believe that one can meaningfully speak of "professional integrity" as distinct from overall moral integrity; and for some issues in bioethics this distinction may be an important one. But we believe that the proper conception of the integrated-self view of integrity for a bioethics consultant cuts across the personal and professional spheres of life. It demands of the ethics consultant a commitment to exemplifying certain moral excellences that express a clearly defined moral identity.

One reason for this is that the good health care ethics consultant is a special sort of teacher whose job is to role-model ethical analysis and reflection. In a typical health care institution, the ethics consultant cannot teach ethics didactically, using terms that people without formal training in ethics may find highly technical and in many ways foreign to their work and experience. Besides, many people in the clinical setting will naturally be more attentive to what the ethics consultant does than to what he says. They will look to see how he behaves and will assume that the behavior they witness is what ethics requires. Thus, an ethics consultant who is obsequious toward physicians but domineering toward nurses is doing a bad job of teaching ethics at his institution. He can hardly be praised as a good ethics consultant, no matter how excellent his reasoning skills in case consultation. To quote one ethicist, "This role calls for circumspection. Bad role modeling by an ethicist can do real damage."[15] Because the ethics consultant's role includes the explicit positive modeling of moral analysis and reflection and the strict avoidance of negative modeling, the ethics consultant differs from others who work in the health care setting and also from the professor of ethics at the university whose job is to teach moral theory.

Further, we suggest that an ethics consultant who adheres to one standard of behavior in his private life and a divergent standard in his professional role is unlikely to model ideal ethical behavior in the way the role requires. To have to stop and think before acting, "Let's see, if I were at home I could lie and cheat, but now I'm at work, so I can't," hardly seems conducive to doing one's duty *in the right way*. And this is quite independent of whether any colleagues in the workplace would ever find out that one is cheating on income tax. A person of integrity has a firm disposition toward acting well even when no one is watching. The income-tax cheat who feels completely comfortable with that behavior, at the same time as working professionally as an ethics consultant, is demonstrating that the consultant need not be a person of integrity. By extension, in his role as an institutional teacher of bioethics, he is telling his colleagues that they need not be persons of integrity in order to be good health care professionals.

An interesting example of this model of integrity is provided by John Lantos in a paper ostensibly about whether lies to children can ever be justified in health care.[16] We say "ostensibly" because the paper in fact may be more about what it means to be a bioethicist. Lantos describes himself staying in a hotel room in a distant city, soon to give a lecture on ethics to a pediatrics research society. He reflects on the white lies he told his children when he left home—he is sorry to have to leave them, but his job demands it. In actuality he enjoys getting away every so often, and these trips are usually elective and not mandatory. Out for an early morning jog, he sees a homeless person sleeping under a statue in the park. Lantos wonders about the hypocrisy of a society that prides itself on being moral by always telling children the truth about a fatal diagnosis but tolerates so many of its citizens having to live in the streets. Now Lantos does not necessarily alter what he will say to his children when he leaves on another trip, nor does he invite the homeless person back to his hotel room. But he thinks about and worries about these things. And he seems to be saying that he worries about them *because* he is a bioethicist.

Good bioethical decision making in a health care setting demands more than blind adherence to rules. It requires thoughtful and deep reflection on values. The good teacher of bioethics will model that sort of thoughtful reflection. The person who lacks integrity often, of necessity, turns off a portion of that reflective function in her life (since such reflection would prove too uncomfortable). We don't think that person will do a good job of modeling good ethical decision making.

Having briefly discussed why character and virtue are central to health care ethics consultation, we now want to discuss the misunderstanding that may have led some ASBH task force members to be uneasy about too much attention to character in the final report. We propose that this unease arises mainly from the distinction between *being* a virtuous person and *proclaiming oneself to be* a virtuous person. Almost always, the latter act reflects something other than true virtue—often the exact opposite. As we suggest above, the virtuous person is more capable than the average individual of discerning how she has fallen short in her quest for virtue. Striving to try harder in the future, not bragging about one's accomplishments, is how persons of real character behave.

This brings us to an unavoidable paradox. The ASBH report is, by its nature, a proclamation of what ethics consultants claim to be. It might be the case, therefore, that ethics consultants ought to be truly persons of good character. But to proclaim this publicly, based on the analysis just given, would seem inevitably to brand us as persons of bad character. So ethics consultants should be virtuous but must never talk about it, especially in task force reports. The inclusion of humility in the list of virtues seems especially to drive this point home: how can one, at the same time, both be humble and proclaim oneself humble? We think this is the main reason that some of our colleagues hesitated to approve the language on character unless it was very carefully circumscribed.

Is there a flaw in this reasoning? The objection to too much attention to character assumes basically one sort of proclamation regarding virtue, one that it is essentially self-congratulatory. Such an act of proclamation presupposes a point-in-time view of virtue—one has, or thinks one has, acquired or achieved virtue at or before the moment of proclamation. But we have argued that this is a wrong-headed account of virtue. True virtue requires a lifetime, biographical account, describing a long-term set of aspirations toward particular moral excellences. Unless the speaker is on her deathbed, a proclamation of having achieved virtue is an admission that one does not understand the concept.

By contrast, while a proclamation of *aspiring to* virtue may have self-serving political implications, it is at least possible that such a proclamation is consistent with a true understanding of what virtue requires. This is especially true if the proclamation includes certain features: the speaker (1) recognizes her current deficiencies, (2) holds herself publicly accountable for her ongoing commitment to developing the desired traits of character, and (3) describes a program by which she can continue to move toward a deeper understanding of those traits and become more successful in exhibiting them. Indeed, if such aspirational proclamations about virtue and character were *not* possible in a manner consistent with the meaning of those concepts, any talk about virtue and character would seem impossible, at least in a practical context. A person should be able to say to his acquaintances that he wishes to be humble and should be able to invite their criticisms of ways in which he presently falls short of humility and what he might do to correct those lapses. And if one person can make such a public statement of aspiration to virtue, then groups such as health care ethics consultants should be able to do so as well. If such a statement (growing out of an honest intention to succeed, or else to be held accountable for failure) is arrogant or self-serving, then it is hard to imagine any effort to be a moral person or to do the morally right thing that is not equally arrogant or self-serving.

In summary, we believe that some of our task force colleagues may have been uneasy about including a robust statement on character in the ASBH report because they feared it would be viewed as arrogant, self-serving, or otherwise unseemly. But this fear is based on confusing a proclamation of having achieved virtue with a proclamation of aspiring to virtue; and on confusing the person who proclaims virtue without possessing it with the person who genuinely wishes to do the hard work necessary to be virtuous over the span of a lifetime.

If this fear is the central concern, then we can see that another objection— that we are somehow claiming that the ethics consultant ought to be *more virtuous* than anyone else in the institution—is really a derivative concern. To claim that virtue and character are central to the role of the health care ethics consultant is not to make any claim about interpersonal comparisons of virtue. Consider the character trait of compassion, for example. It may well be that the caregivers who directly treat the sick have, and display, much more compassion than the ethics consultant. But these care providers are not expected, as a necessary part of their role, to be especially articulate about what compassion consists of or requires, nor are they especially supposed to be role models of compassion for others. By contrast, as a teacher of ethics within the institution, the ethics consultant is expected to be able to describe and to model compassionate behavior sufficiently for others to grasp the nature and scope of that virtue clearly. Also, the ethics consultant is expected to take compassion seriously and (at the very least) to avoid any obvious lack of compassion in the way she treats all the personnel, patients, and families with whom she interacts. Thus, saying that character is more central to the consultant's role is hardly to say anything at all about how much or how little of a particular character trait the ethics consultant possesses, compared with any other worker.

For all these reasons, we do not merely defend the language on character included in the ASBH report; we maintain that it could, with profit, have been even further developed and expanded, perhaps with particular attention to the distinction between personal and social virtues.

Whose Virtue? Which Character?

MARK P. AULISIO, DAN W. BROCK, AND WILLIAM WINSLADE

In the first part of this chapter, Françoise Baylis and Howard Brody argue for the importance of good character, or virtue, for health care ethics consultants. For our part, we do not intend to argue that good character is unimportant for ethics consultants; that ethics consultants, or anyone else, should lack courage, integrity, or some other virtue. Saying that ethics consultants should strive to be virtuous or should have courage or integrity, for example, is noncontroversial. However, if being "virtuous" or having "courage" or "integrity" is going to add something meaningful to the role for ethics consultation articulated in the ASBH report, a great deal more will have to be said. The more that must be said, however, the more profoundly problematic the discussion becomes. Our concern, then, is not so much with the claim that ethics consultants should have good character or be virtuous (we think everyone should strive to be virtuous) as with the notoriously problematic nature of these concepts and what is necessary for them to add something substantive to the role for ethics consultation, with its attendant knowledge and skills, as laid out in the ASBH report.

If the concept of character, or character "traits," is to add anything meaningful to the role for ethics consultation, and to the related skills and knowledge put forth in the ASBH report, then it will need to be defined. As suggested by the passage from the report quoted at the beginning of this chapter, this is no trivial task. Whether "character" is an observable behavior or set of behaviors, a disposition to behave in certain ways, or something else, is important for a host of related issues, including: whether and how "character" might be taught or modeled, whether and how "character" might be tested, whether "character" is pervasive throughout personality and behavior or whether it can be compartmentalized, and so forth.

If character is defined, for example, as observable behavior in a given domain, it is very difficult to see what a discussion of it will add to the role for ethics consultation with its attendant skills and knowledge, as articulated in the ASBH report. In practice, carrying out the role well and properly *just will be* what it means for an ethics consultant to have the requisite "character." Similarly, suppose the claim regarding character is stronger, that is, character is something more, something that goes beyond behavior—as in the traditional notion of "virtue" as a more global *habitus* or "disposition to behave" in certain ways.[17] Absent a robust conception of human nature, notion of the good, and related philosophical psychology, it is still difficult to see what the discussion will add. If certain dispositions are necessary for the development of certain skills or for behaving in certain ways, then those without the requisite *habitus* will simply be unable to develop the requisite skills necessary to the role of ethics consultation. Here, too, the discussion of "character" does not seem to add much to the discussion of the role of ethics consultation, and the attendant skills and knowledge needed to carry out that role, at least as characterized in the ASBH report.

To be sure, when Baylis, Brody, and others discuss the importance of character for ethics consultation, they clearly both intend to and do add substance to the conversation about ethics consultation, as the following passage indicates (emphasis added):

> It may well be that the caregivers who directly treat the sick have, and display, much more compassion than the ethics consultant. *But these care providers are not expected, as a necessary part of their role, to be especially articulate about what compassion consists of or requires, nor are they especially supposed to be role models of compassion for others. By contrast, as a teacher of ethics within the institution, the ethics consultant is expected to be able to describe and to model compassionate behavior sufficiently for others to grasp the nature and scope of that virtue clearly.* Also, the ethics consultant is expected to take compassion seriously, and (at the very least) to avoid any obvious lack of compassion in the way she treats all the personnel, patients, and families with whom she interacts. Thus, saying that *character is more central to the consultant's role* is hardly to say anything at all about how much or how little of a particular character trait the ethics consultant possesses, compared with any other worker.

In giving ethics consultants the role of being exemplars or role models of certain types of virtue, this passage goes well beyond the role of ethics consultation characterized in the ASBH report. Character is, of course, central to being an exemplar or role model of virtue, but here *character* necessarily appeals to a robust substantive notion of the good. This view casts the role of ethics consultant in the vein of hero, sage, guru, imam, or mahatma—Aristotle's "great souled" to whom others look for meaning and guidance in life.[18]

Though we agree that all who do ethics consultation should strive to be good people—to be virtuous—we do not think health professionals, patients, or surrogates should look to ethics consultants as role models or exemplars of virtue; nor do we think ethics consultants should view themselves as having the role of modeling virtue so that others can learn how to be good persons. Rather, ethics consultants, as the ASBH report suggests, should be present for the purpose of helping to identify and analyze value conflicts or uncertainties that inevitably come up in today's health care environment and attempting to facilitate acceptable resolutions of those value conflicts or uncertainties, given the context that gives rise to them in the first place.

We understand that some may look at ethics consultants as exemplars or models of virtue, but we do not think this is a role ethics consultants should have or encourage. Such a view would dramatically expand the consultant's role beyond that characterized in the ASBH report and is arguably inconsistent with it. Expanding consultants' role to include exemplar or role model of virtue bestows on them a profound authority and expertise. Indeed, such an expansion of consultants' role implies that ethics consultants *qua* ethics consultants must have a privileged conception of the good and a special excellence in living the good life. This is deeply problematic for many reasons, only a few of which we consider here.

Expanding the consultant's role to include being a role model for virtuous living raises the profound question of whose conception of the good should ground the operative concept of virtue. Adapting the title *Whose Justice? Which Rationality?* of the famous work by Alasdair MacIntyre,[19] we ask: *Whose virtue? Which character?*

Shusako Endo, in his provocative novel *Silence,* describes a young man who became a Catholic priest and then went off to convert the "heathen" in Japan.[20] Thanks to the success of missionaries who had gone before him, Catholicism was steadily growing. With its growth came violent suppression, as missionaries and converts alike were brutally tortured and martyred. Endo portrays the young priest as determined to shed his blood for the faith, should he be put to the test. After converting thousands, he is captured and asked to renounce his faith or watch hundreds of his converts be tortured and killed. What does virtue require? What would the courageous person, the person of integrity, do? Endo's young priest renounces his faith and his converts are spared. Was he courageous or cowardly, a man of integrity or dissolution, a saint or a sinner?

A poor father of twelve struggled with whether to give up his job as manager at a convenience store, because it sold magazines that were "an occasion of sin" for patrons of the store. At the time, unemployment in his county was at 22 percent. Before quitting his job, he petitioned the store to stop selling the magazines, but to no avail. He quit his job because he decided that he could no longer be party to the evil being perpetrated by the convenience store chain. Was he virtuous, courageous, and of great integrity, or irresponsible, self-righteous, and prideful?

As Baylis and Brody point out, some of the task force discussions centered on whether one could be a good ethics consultant and cheat on one's income tax. They use this example as a lead-in to discussing integrity and critiquing the view that "character" can be compartmentalized between "private," "professional," and other spheres. This example, however, lends itself well to the concern here. Suppose, for example, that the "cheating" was in protest of the death penalty, nuclear proliferation, or the use of public funds for abortion. Just as with the examples offered above, depending on one's conception of the good, this might be either virtuous or vicious.

Finally, the profound problem of adjudicating among conceptions of the good is formidable enough in its own right, but considering it in terms of the role of ethics consultants adds layers of complexity. Over time, all individuals work out their own conception of the good, their own set of values by which they choose to live. Furthermore, all citizens in our society have a right to their own set of values and, within certain limits, to live their life accordingly. This right extends to all involved in health care ethics consultation in our society, be they ethics consultants and health professionals or patients, family members, and surrogates. Extending the role of ethics consultants to include being exemplars or role models of virtue is deeply problematic in the light of these rights. On the one hand, patients, surrogates, and health care providers should not have to look to ethics consultants as role models of virtue, as if an ethics consultant's view of the good life should be privileged with any special normative weight. On the other hand, ethics consultants should not seek to promote their own view of the good as if it were privileged: on the contrary, they should discourage this, because it risks eroding the decision-making authority of legitimate decision makers in particular cases. Indeed, actively promoting one's own view of the good could easily lead to consultants overstepping their bounds and subtly (or not so subtly) imposing their values on involved parties; such an imposition is fundamentally inconsistent with the role of ethics consultation characterized in the ASBH report. As such, not only is expanding the ethics consultant's role to include being a role model of good character or exemplar of virtue not part of the role for ethics consultation laid out in the ASBH report, but it actually threatens to undermine that role.

Conclusion: "But There Is *Some* Common Ground"

As the two parts of this chapter make clear, there is strong disagreement about the nature and importance of good character for ethics consultants in their role as ethics consultant. These differences mark what will undoubtedly be an on-going debate in the field. Should ethics consultants be expected to be role models of virtue for others in health care? Should they be "expected to be able to describe and to model" virtuous behavior "sufficiently for others to grasp the nature and scope" of certain virtues? Or, conversely, does such a view at best add little to, and at worst threaten to undermine, the legitimate role for health care ethics consultation as laid out in the ASBH report?

In closing, we wish to underscore a point on which there is no dispute: those who do ethics consultation, like all others in health care (and all other areas of life), should strive to be of good character, to be virtuous. But exactly, or even roughly, what this means and how it adds to the discussion of health care ethics consultation is, as we have seen, a matter of some dispute.

Notes

1. Society for Health and Human Values–Society for Bioethics Consultation: Task Force on Standards for Bioethics Consultation, *Core Competencies for Health Care Ethics Consultation: The Report of the American Society for Bioethics and Humanities* (Glenview, Ill.: American Society for Bioethics and Humanities, 1998), pp. 21–22.

2. Freedman, B., *Duty and Healing: Foundations of a Jewish Bioethic* (New York: Routledge, 1999), p. 69. For Benjamin Freedman, the duty perspective is grounded in a Jewish approach to bioethics, but justifications for this approach can also be found in other religious and secular ethical systems.

3. Ibid., p. 127.

4. Ibid., p. 55.

5. Baylis, F., "Health Care Ethics Consultation: 'Training in Virtue,'" *Human Studies* 22, no. 1 (1999):26.

6. ASBH report, pp. 21–23.

7. Freedman, B., "Where Are the Heroes of Bioethics?" *Journal of Clinical Ethics* 7, no. 4 (1996):298.

8. Andre, J., "Speaking Truth to Employers," *Journal of Clinical Ethics* 8, no. 2 (1997):199–203.

9. Baylis, F., "A Profile of the Health Care Ethics Consultant," in *The Health Care Ethics Consultant*, ed. F. Baylis (Totowa, N.J.: Humana Press, 1994), p. 38.

10. Calhoun, C., "Standing for Something," *Journal of Philosophy* 92, no. 5 (1995):252, 259.

11. Benjamin, M., *Splitting the Difference: Compromise and Integrity in Ethics and Politics* (Lawrence, Kans.: University Press of Kansas, 1990); Calhoun, "Standing for Something."

12. Webster, G., and Baylis, F., "Moral Residue," in *Margin of Error: The Necessity,*

Inevitability, and Ethics of Mistakes in Medicine and Bioethics Consultation, ed. S. Rubin and L. Zoloth (Hagerstown, Md.: University Publishing Group, 1999).

13. Calhoun, "Standing for Something," p. 254.

14. This idea was initially put forward for discussion by Paul Schyve, a member of the ASBH task force.

15. Andre, "Speaking Truth to Employers," p. 200.

16. Lantos, J.D., "Should We Always Tell Children the Truth?" *Perspectives in Biology and Medicine* 40, no. 1 (1996):78–92.

17. MacIntyre, A., *After Virtue* (Notre Dame, Ind.: University of Notre Dame Press, 1981).

18. Freedman, "Where Are the Heroes of Bioethics?"

19. MacIntyre, A., *Whose Justice? Which Rationality?* (Notre Dame, Ind.: University of Notre Dame Press, 1988).

20. Endo, S., *Silence,* trans. W. Johnston (Tokyo: Sophia University and C.E. Tuttle, 1969).

II • PRACTICAL QUESTIONS

4

Innovative Educational Programs

A Necessary First Step toward Improving Quality in Ethics Consultation

JACQUELINE J. GLOVER, PH.D., AND WILLIAM NELSON, PH.D.

During the past two decades, ethics consultations in health care have been increasingly recognized as an important resource for patients, families, clinicians, and hospital management.[1] Ethics consultations may address complex ethical, psychosocial, and spiritual issues that can directly affect patient care or influence an institution's policy or procedures. Members of ethics committees frequently provide ethics consultations, but rarely do they have formal training in applied ethics. Because of the potential influence of ethics consultation on patient care, many people are debating the scope of education or training that ethics consultants should receive.[2] This call for an intentional look at the educational needs of ethics consultants led to the formation of the Task Force on Standards for Bioethics Consultation and publication of its report, *Core Competencies for Health Care Ethics Consultation.*[3] Some ethics consultants are also recognizing their need for continuing education to meet the ever-expanding list of clinical and organizational ethical challenges.[4] These factors have encouraged ethics educators and consultants to develop and seek out ethics education programs.

Ethics consultations may be performed by a variety of health care professionals and community members. What specific training should these individuals possess to function effectively as an ethics consultant? Whether consultation is provided by an individual, a small team of professionals, or an ethics committee, competent consultants are essential. As noted in the ASBH report, "patients, families, surrogates, and health care providers deserve assurance that when they seek help sorting through the ethical dimensions of health care, ethics consultants are competent to offer that assistance. Given the nature and goals of ethics consultation . . . we believe consultants must possess certain skills, knowledge, and character traits to perform competently."[5] The specific skills, knowledge, and character traits required are delineated in the report.

We accept the premise that all ethics consultants need at least the basic skills and knowledge as presented in the report. Where ethics consultations are done by an individual, she or he should possess a higher level of skills and knowledge. All health care professionals or community members performing ethics consultations should review their skills and knowledge in the light of the ASBH report. Some programs, including that of the West Virginia Network of Ethics Committees, have developed a specialized self-assessment form that ethics consultants can use to gauge their strengths and weaknesses and assess areas that need further education and skill-building experiences. When knowledge and skills require improvement, health care professionals and community members should seek continuing education to fill the need. This benefits not only the ethics consultant but also the institution being served.

Meeting the educational needs of ethics consultants is complicated by the reality of limited time and money, which creates challenges for both ethics consultants and their institutions. However, if the institution's leadership acknowledges the importance of having a good ethics consultation service to enhance patient care and organizational decision making and ensuring quality in the work of ethics consultants, then the administration should provide release time and financial support to allow ethics consultants to participate in educational opportunities.

In this chapter we discuss various models and methods whereby ethics consultants can increase their skills and knowledge, which we believe is crucial for improving the overall quality of ethics consultations. We describe both traditional programs and innovative programs that use modern education technology to foster learning. The various programs described here are meant only as examples of the various possibilities, not as an exhaustive list of the resources available, nor as a prescriptive model of what educational programs must be like. Whatever educational method is employed, the goals and objectives should seek to help the consultant acquire the recommended knowledge and skills and reinforce the appropriate character traits for ethics consultation.

Most education for ethics consultation occurs in settings outside formal degree programs. These settings range from informal self-study to programs offered by individual ethics committees, ethics centers, regional networks of ethics committees, independent ethics consultants, and ethics resources such as the National Center for Ethics in Health Care of the Veterans Health Administration (VHA). We assume that few ethics consultants have the time or resources to enter formal degree programs. Where this is possible, health care professionals and others should explore the many university-based opportunities. Also, since individuals and committees rarely have the resources to sponsor ongoing and in-depth training in ethics consultation, our discussion focuses on the various educational models used by regional centers, networks, independent consultants, and health care systems. At best, these organizations function in alliance with individual ethics committees and/or ethics consultants to provide training materials and continuing support.

Whichever educational model is chosen, it must strive to meet all three components of the core competencies: knowledge, skills, and character. Knowledge is perhaps the easiest component. We are all familiar with the usual methods for presenting the basic content areas in bioethics—some combination of lecture and case- or issue-driven discussion. Skill building is more challenging, requiring creative use of interactive discussion, modeling, and role-playing.

The character component is perhaps the most difficult. The ASBH task force struggled long and hard over the importance of the ethics consultant's character in relation to performing consultations, concluding that a consultant's character "is important for optimal ethics consultation." But some have suggested that you cannot teach character and cannot screen ethics consultants for character. These challenges have important implications for the training of ethics consultants. Rather than ignoring the important issues associated with character, we believe these issues must be acknowledged and discussed in educational programs. Possible subjects for discussion include the correlation between character and the quality of ethics consultation; what character means and what key characteristics are necessary for consultation; how the concept of character can be applied in the selection of ethics consultants; and how character can be nurtured within the context of an ethics committee or a group of ethics consultants. Adding a question about the character of the individuals involved, including the consultant, can be a useful part of any case discussion. In our experience, the best way to "teach" character is through mentoring programs. Witnessing a role model exhibiting the essential character traits, then reflecting with the mentor about how these character traits influence the consultation process, is a very powerful teaching method.

Ethics committee members who perform ethics consultations have the responsibility for self-development. Every ethics committee should have an initial training period as it is getting started, which should last from several months to a year, depending on the frequency of meetings. Before an ethics committee starts performing consultations, team members should receive a thorough orientation in the basic knowledge, skills, and character traits discussed in the ASBH report. Equally important is the availability of an orientation process for new members as they join the committee. Ethics committees are also required to provide ongoing discussion of substantive issues in health care ethics and the process of ethics consultation. Some kind of manual or similar resource is very valuable. A manual developed for the West Virginia University Hospitals Ethics Committee includes a copy of the history of the committee; a list of current members; copies of various informational items about the committee that are used to advertise the committee at the institution (e.g., patient information brochures and articles from the medical staff news-letter or house staff manuals); various consultation tools (summary of the consultation process, sample consultation notes, format for a patient care con-ference, evaluation tools); relevant institutional policies; relevant state legis-lation; and selected articles and a bibliography for further reading. One or two articles in each of the knowledge areas, as well as articles about communication and negotiation skills, are essential.

It is the rare committee that can develop and sustain a robust educational program on its own. Many ethics committees regularly sponsor educational programs for their members and the entire health care institution. Other com-mittees offer a full-day retreat for ethics committee members to keep up with current issues and sharpen their consultation tools. Most committees turn to outside sources to help in these educational efforts or to provide workshops for their members.

In general, there are five forms of educational activities for ethics committee members:

1. face-to-face programs of varying lengths;
2. extended educational programs;
3. distance-learning methodologies such as web-based courses, CD-ROMs, and video or telephone conferences;
4. fellowships, certificates, and degree programs; and
5. ongoing support or mentoring from regional networks, centers, or inde-pendent consultants.

We cannot overemphasize the importance of these resources as ethics commit-tees around the country experience common challenges, including the move-ment from an inpatient-focused to an outpatient-focused health care system, the addition of an organizational ethics focus, and a growing recognition that ethics committee members are overburdened and undereducated.

Face-to-Face Educational Programs

The most common educational activity is participation in face-to-face educational programs, which can range from small seminars to large conferences and can last from one hour to several days. Some programs even have multiple components that extend over a long period of time. Face-to-face programs have the advantage of reinforcing learning through group and interactive processes and providing opportunities for networking with colleagues and group or team building. Off-site face-to-face education can involve expensive travel, time away from the workplace, and difficulty in reproducing the experience for other learners. Despite some disadvantages, however, it continues to be an effective learning strategy, particularly for the development of new skills.[6]

Daylong Programs

Many ethics centers, independent ethics consultants, and regional ethics committee networks offer daylong programs on the basics of ethics consultation that combine a lecture format with small-group discussion of cases. Many, like the one offered by the Department of Bioethics at The Cleveland Clinic Foundation in November 1999, begin with an introduction to the core concepts of ethical decision making (40 minutes); the basic who, what, where, and when of ethics consultation (30 minutes); and the process of ethics consultation (30 minutes). This is followed by 90-minute break-out sessions for small groups to go through various ethics consultation cases. The afternoon is spent on such nuts and bolts issues as charting and follow-up (30 minutes), evaluation of ethics consultations (30 minutes), and an interactive session of a mock consultation process (60 minutes). The daylong program uses three faculty members, is about eight and one-half hours in length, and costs between $90 and $150, depending on participants' affiliation with the sponsoring organization.

The daylong workshop format is well suited to covering common bioethical issues and concepts as articulated in the ASBH report. Most ethics centers and regional ethics networks offer such workshops several times a year. These workshops are also well suited to the combination of lecture and small-group case discussion. Presentations that link the subject matter directly to consultation, possibly through the use of illustrative cases, are more effective in preparing ethics consultants for their work. An interactive discussion of a case by a multidisciplinary panel can be very effective.

Three- to Four-Day Programs

Many ethics centers and regional networks have offered special extended programs devoted specifically to training in the core competencies. The summer program conducted by the West Virginia Network of Ethics Committees in 1998 is one example.[7] The program lasted three days, with twenty formal in-session hours. It was held at a resort where people could spend time together networking and sharing resources. The program was designed as a train-the-trainer workshop, providing participants with a book of resources for the training of their ethics committees and discussing the best ways to teach the subject matter in their own settings.

All participants received a mailed preconference self-assessment form to help them determine their strengths and weaknesses and provide input into the conference content. The conference began with a summary of the results of the self-assessments and a pretest, in which the 125 or so participants divided into multidisciplinary consultation teams of three or four and worked through an initial ethics consultation. This pretest case was then used in an initial interactive session to identify the core knowledge and skills. Other presentations (45 to 60 minutes each) included the use of moral theory, the process of ethics consultation, the role of character, assessing decision-making capacity, withholding and withdrawing treatment, West Virginia legislation, medical futility, organizational ethics, and risk-management issues in ethics consultations. Most of these presentations were followed by an hour of small-group discussion of cases. Some innovative sessions included an interactive panel of faculty talking about key interpersonal skills and role-playing examples, a panel of faculty members talking about mistakes they had made and how to avoid them, and a session on how to evaluate the level of core competencies of ethics committee members.

The workshop concluded with a post-test that followed the same format as the pretest, three to four multidisciplinary team members working through an ethics consultation. These post-tests were "graded" by faculty, and the results were reported to participants in a letter they could add to their certificate of attendance as evidence of training in the core competencies.

This three-day program attracted participants from different disciplines, used four faculty members, and cost about $300 for members of the West Virginia Network of Ethics Committees and $350 for nonmembers, plus room and board.

Four- to Five-Day Programs

Several ethics centers sponsor four- to five-day ethics courses such as "Intensive Training Course: Practical Knowledge and Skills for Building an Effective Ethics Program," offered by the VHA's National Center for Ethics in Health Care.[8] This four-day intensive course is designed to provide a select group of a hundred ethics program leaders within VHA—including administrators, clinicians, and members of ethics advisory committees—with specialized knowledge and skills to improve the effectiveness of their hospital ethics programs. The course emphasizes the practical knowledge, skills, and character that those serving as ethics resources will need to create "integrated ethics programs." An integrated ethics program is a systematic issues-oriented approach to improving an institution's ethics practices and quality of care; it is a newly conceived way of anticipating and responding to recurring ethical issues. The National Center for Ethics in Health Care sees it as the logical next step in the evolution of ethics advisory committees. As in the traditional ethics committee, members must acquire and develop their knowledge and skills to promote and clarify ethical standards of practice. The course explores the barriers to a successful ethics program and describes strategies for improving the effectiveness and coordination of the various components of an institution's ethics service, including the ethics committee, compliance office, legal counsel, business office, information management, and institutional review boards.

Each day of the program includes didactic presentations, small-group case studies or exercises, and large-group discussions addressing the following practical topics:

- building of an integrated ethics program;
- application of a results-oriented approach to ethical problem solving;
- moral reasoning and ethical analysis;
- clinical, organizational, and research ethics issues and concepts;
- process and interpersonal skills for ethics advisory committee members;
- ways to overcome barriers to a successful ethics program;
- evaluation and assessment of ethics activities; and
- development of local plans to achieve an integrated ethics program and the core competencies outlined in the ASBH report.

The *knowledge* aspect of the curriculum is provided mainly through lecture or panel presentations. Each faculty member accompanies his or her presentation with PowerPoint material and creates an interactive learning experience. The PowerPoint presentations are also posted on the center's web site (www.va.gov/vhaethics). The course's educational strategy is to create an environment that gives participants constant opportunities to interact with faculty and with other learners to gain practical and relevant knowledge and skills to enhance their ethics program.[9] Acquiring the necessary skills for problem solving or case consultation requires learning by "doing." Throughout the week, participants practice their skills in small groups. The case- or issue-driven groups practice addressing ethical issues, with feedback from an experienced ethics consultant. The cases and issues are written to generate questions about processes for performing ethical analyses. The issue-oriented discussions focus on the creation of ethical standards of practice to prevent ethical conflicts. This quality-management approach to ethics seeks to promote and clarify ethical standards and practices. The course participants receive extensive resource materials to expand their learning experience and to provide resources for local educational activities.

Extended Educational Programs

Some regional centers have developed extended curricula to help train participating institutions in the core competencies. For example, the University of Pittsburgh's Consortium Ethics Program sponsors a regular three-year basic and advanced ethics curriculum and site visits for ethics committee members and ethics consultants at the program's forty-five participating institutions. The three-year curriculum is structured roughly as follows:

- year 1: "Ethics and Clinical Practice" (exploring basic issues in bioethics)
- year 2: "Law and Health Care Ethics" (fundamental legal issues in bioethics for the basic group and special issues in law and bioethics for the advanced group)
- year 3: "The Humanities and Bioethics" (contributions of literature, history, and philosophy to health care and bioethics)

Typically, the Consortium Ethics Program curriculum consists of five to seven sessions in each track per year, along with a weekend intensive retreat modeled much like the three-day programs described above. Staff members also make site visits to the participating institutions (about 100 to 130 visits per year), educating ethics committee members and staff on specific issues particular to that institution and concentrating on building the skills necessary for ethics consultation.

The program includes special sessions on ethics consultation processes and evaluation for both the basic and advanced groups. One session focuses on the "ethics facilitation" approach to ethics consultation described in the ASBH report, and another focuses on medical futility. All the sessions are germane to the core competencies, because they address the knowledge and skills articulated in the report. Other sessions address the role of character in ethics consultation, including the session "Ethics Consultation and the Preservation of Integrity."

Some sessions are worth highlighting here, because they go beyond the standard "basic issues in bioethics"—informed consent, confidentiality, decision-making capacity, and end-of-life decision making—that one should expect from any basic continuing education curriculum in bioethics. One session deals with informed consent and delivering bad news. After faculty members model discussions that went well and poorly, class participants role-play difficult scenarios. This is an excellent way to build skills in listening and communication. The session "End of Life Decisions: An Islamic Perspective" addresses the need for knowledge of religious and cultural perspectives. "Creating a Common Ethic for Health Care" focuses on justice issues in health care.

Each session typically lasts four hours, with lunch, and offers 3.0 continuing medical education (CME) credits. The registration fee is $20 for Consortium Ethics Program representatives and $60 for others. There is an institutional membership fee for the Consortium Ethics Program.

Another educational model involves the development of a specialized curriculum for an individual ethics committee. The Bioethics Network of Ohio (known as BENO) offers a ten-session yearlong program to help health care organizations establish and develop ethics committees. Each session is approximately 90 minutes long.

The core curriculum consists of seven sessions: "Clinical Ethics" (two sessions), "End-of-Life Issues" (two sessions), "Decisional Capacity," "Law and Ethics," and "Case Consultation." In addition to these core sessions, the ethics committee can choose from a list of electives for the remaining three sessions. Options for the elective sessions include the topics continuity of care, religion and bioethics, rationing/managed care, culture of health care, caregiver ethics, and one "open" session on a topic specific to the ethics committee's needs. Longer workshops are also offered on the subject of educational activities by ethics committees, policy writing and review, and applied case consultation. At the close of the yearlong program, a BENO-sponsored faculty member is available for an extended committee retreat to help in a strategic planning session for the future of the committee. This model is quite expensive, with the ten-session curriculum, the workshops, and the retreat priced separately.

Distance Learning

Ethics education has historically been conducted either through face-to-face activities or through self-teaching, by reading the ethics literature. However, both educators and learners should consider alternatives. After clearly determining their educational goals and objectives, educators should carefully assess what method of providing education is most likely to achieve the goals in a manner that is both accessible to learners and cost-effective. Educators can no longer assume that face-to-face teaching methods are the most appropriate. Some alternatives include print materials, satellite broadcasts, videotapes, CD-ROMs (electronic publishing and interactive courses), web-based training and publishing, audioconferencing, videoconferencing, and email. Each delivery method has its advantages and limitations for both the educator and the learner, and selecting the most appropriate method depends on both parties. We highlight a few examples of distance-learning methods that have proved effective.

Web-Based Courses

Michigan State University, in East Lansing, has offered web courses, and the Center for the Study of Bioethics at the Medical College of Wisconsin, in Milwaukee, is currently offering web courses in bioethics.

The Michigan State University course, a fifteen-week curriculum titled "Issues in Health Care Ethics," focuses on ethical issues most commonly brought to institutional ethics committees. The emphasis is on developing the background knowledge and skills needed to critically analyze and assess normative positions taken on ethical issues. One of the course's objectives is to develop the skills necessary to function effectively as an ethics committee member. These skills include the abilities to identify ethical issues in health care and discuss them in a thoughtful, informed, and respectful manner; to critically assess arguments and positions on ethical issues; and to articulate positions on ethical issues carefully and clearly.

The participants have reading assignments, participate in online discussions, and write short reaction papers responding to these assignments and discussions. Each participant is also required to complete an integrative project on a chosen topic, preferably related to some work on an ethics committee or in a health care institution. Information about the course is available on the university's web site (www.vu.msu.edu/preview/ost590/index.html).

The course was offered either for three hours of academic credit or for twenty-five hours of CME credit in its first year, fifty hours of CME credit in its second year. The cost was $660 for academic credit and $800 for CME credit. Academic credit was offered either as a medical college course or as a humanities course, according to the needs of the participant.

The web courses at the Medical College of Wisconsin are offered as part of a certificate program in clinical bioethics or an executive-style M.A. in bioethics. Both programs attract participants from across the nation and around the world. Information is available on the college's web site (www.mcw.edu/bioethics/).

The certificate in clinical bioethics is designed to provide a basic introduction to the philosophical, legal, and clinical foundations of health care ethics, to enhance the clinical practice of health care professionals, and/or to provide a foundation for further study for such professionals or academics. The program consists of four courses: "Philosophical Bioethics" (3 credits), "Clinical Topics in Bioethics" (2 credits), "Law and Bioethics" (2 credits), and "Justice and Healthcare" (2 credits). Two courses are usually offered in each of the fall and spring semesters. In addition to graduate credit, participants can also earn CME credits (50 category 1 credits per course) and continuing education credit for other health care professionals. All graduate credits are applicable toward the college's M.A. degree.

The executive-style M.A. in bioethics provides advanced training for professionals who wish to prepare for teaching, research, policy development, and clinical work related to bioethics. The program includes didactic, clinical, and research components, and culminates in the student's presentation of a master's thesis project. The program has two components: (1) a large number of courses delivered by web-based and other distance-education formats, and (2) one intensive three-week summer session on the college campus. Courses available in the distance-education formats include "Clinical Topics in Bioethics" (2 credits), "Justice and Healthcare" (2 credits), "Law and Bioethics" (2 credits), "Philosophical Bioethics" (3 credits), "Ethics of Medical Informatics" (1.5 credits), "Epidemiology" (3 credits), "Ethics of Healthcare Technologies" (1.5 credits), "Readings and Research" (3 credits), and "Master's Thesis" (6 credits).

The advantages of web-based programs are obvious. They attract participants from a wide geographic area who would not ordinarily have access to such programs. Class discussions and case analyses are conducted in non-real time, so students can participate at their own pace and convenience during each week. The technical requirements are minimal for these web-based courses—ability to use a web browser and email. The pedagogical capabilities of the web environment enhance the "class" discussions through access to other resources and through individualized instructor feedback. These courses empower learners to find resources and are truly student-centered.

Web courses have some drawbacks, however. First, they are very labor intensive for the faculty: in a sense, the instructor is never out of the classroom. Students log on at all hours, often with direct questions for the faculty. Keeping up with class discussion takes time and diligence. Second, these courses are necessarily geared toward knowledge content and certain analytical skills. Other, more hands-on skills associated with ethics consultations, such as interviewing patients and families and facilitating discussions at patient care or ethics committee meetings, must be acquired elsewhere.

Other Web-Based Resources

Most ethics centers and regional networks of ethics committees have a web site that serves as a type of continuing support for constituents. The typical web page includes general information about the center or network, a calendar of events, direct links to faculty email, links to other ethics sites and resources, and links to relevant state-legislation sites. Many web sites are beginning to include other types of resources so as to increase access to materials formerly available only in printed form. Examples include various tools for ethics consultation, such as a summary of the consultation process and a sample consultation note; evaluation forms for staff and families; and sample institutional policies. Annotated bibliographies of key articles are also very helpful. Many web pages include cases for discussion, and a few provide the opportunity to discuss the cases online.

An innovative program is being offered by the MCP Hahnemann University School of Medicine. "MedEthEx Online: Computer Assisted Instruction in Medical Ethics and Communication Skills on the World Wide Web" (http://griffin.mcphu.edu/medethex/) is a multimedia, case-focused, computer-based learning program in medical ethics and communication skills, free to all users. It gives learners an opportunity to focus on ethical issues in patient care by interacting with a simulated patient. MedEthEx Online was developed to augment courses in medical ethics and training in clinical skills, and it is designed to help bridge the gap between what is taught in the classroom and what happens at the bedside. The program is free to users on the web. It has been used successfully by more than four hundred medical students, and ethics consultants may also benefit from this interactive program.

CD-ROM

VHA has developed a CD-ROM, *Ethics Advisory Committee Resource Material,* which includes articles about the basic knowledge and skills required for ethics consultation, video case studies, VHA ethics-related policies, and an extensive bibliography. This educational resource, compact and portable, is a comprehensive and readily available source of information for ethics advisory committee members.

Though the CD-ROM has been well received and frequently used as an educational resource, it has some major drawbacks. It was labor intensive and expensive to create and, unlike web-based resources, is not easily updated.

Audioconferencing and Videoconferencing

Audioconferencing (telephone conferencing) is a simple yet effective way to reach a wide audience of learners. It is particularly effective in presenting new material, such as a new policy. VHA's National Center for Ethics in Health Care hosts monthly telephone conference calls to all Department of Veterans Affairs ethics advisory committees and ethics leaders, to share information, explore specific ethics issues, and encourage networking among those involved in ethics programs. This series has been conducted since late 2000 and averages more than seventy-five call-in lines and several hundred participants per call. Detailed transcripts are made available on the VHA's Intranet.

Videoconferencing is a cost-effective interactive learning strategy. Printed materials can be sent out to complement the videoconference. Many ethics centers, including VHA's National Center for Ethics in Health Care, also have access to videoconferencing capabilities. This is an excellent way for a center's faculty to join with local ethics committees for a case discussion or discussion of a specific issue that has been identified for further education.

Like all educational activities, audioconferencing and videoconferencing require a clear set of educational goals, careful planning to avoid technical problems, and presenters that interact well with learners and achieve the conferences' intended goals.

Fellowships, Certificates, and Degree Programs

The number of graduate programs offering fellowships, certificates, and degree programs in bioethics/humanities has increased about 182 percent since 1990. According to a 2001 report *North American Graduate Bioethics and Medical Humanities Training Program Survey*, available from the ASBH,[10] there are now forty-seven institutions offering a total of 104 programs: 62 master's degree programs, 13 fellowship programs, 11 certificate programs, and 1 program of individual advanced training (not leading to a certificate, fellowship, or degree). A fuller description of these programs is available in the ASBH survey report or on individual institutional web sites.

Institutions offering certificate programs include (by region): Drew University, Duquesne University, Montefiore Medical Center, Cleveland State University, Medical College of Wisconsin, The University of Chicago, Youngstown State University, Midwestern University, Loma Linda University, and University of Washington. Institutions or organizations offering fellowships include: The University of British Columbia, University of Pennsylvania, University of Pittsburgh, American Medical Association, The Cleveland Clinic, The University of Chicago, University of Wisconsin–Milwaukee, Georgetown University, the Johns Hopkins University, National Institutes of Health, and University of Texas M. D. Anderson Cancer Center.

As the number of opportunities to pursue fellowships, certificates, and degrees increases, we can expect increasing numbers of ethics consultants to undergo this training. We recognize, however, that it is increasingly difficult for many ethics consultants to find the time and the resources to take advantage of such opportunities, and we believe that although this training is desirable, it is not mandatory.

Continuing Support and Mentoring

Ethics centers, regional networks of ethics committees, and independent ethics consultants often work to provide continuing support to people doing ethics consultation. Not only do they serve as a central resource for continuing education through newsletters, web pages, speaker's bureaus, workshops, and other educational opportunities, but they also can provide timely advice in difficult cases. The quality of ethics consultation is enhanced by consultants sharing resources and linking together to discuss difficult issues and cases.

Evaluation

The final issue important to our discussion is the necessity for evaluation, which is essential for continuous quality improvement of ethics consultations.[11] Evaluation has several components. One is an evaluation of whether educational programs are meeting their objectives and the needs of their participants. Another is the direct evaluation of the ethics consultation itself. Most ethics centers have copies of various evaluation tools being used by local ethics consultants. It is important to get evaluations from institutional staff and also, where appropriate, from patients and families.[12]

The final and most difficult component is evaluation of the ethics consultants themselves. Attending educational programs is vastly different from demonstrating a competence in performing ethics consultations. Various programs with a pretest and post-test format, or a mentoring format in which experienced ethics consultants work with trainees, are struggling to bridge that gap. The entire notion of developing residency programs and/or certifying exams is fraught with difficulties. But as the bioethics and health care communities take quality improvement in ethics consultation more seriously, models for demonstrating and documenting the competence of ethics consultants will emerge. It is not hard to imagine that some day the Joint Commission on Accreditation of Healthcare Organizations will look for documentation of competence in ethics consultations as well as some positive outcomes from the process. Some initial ideas include developing a file on each ethics committee member doing consultations or on each individual ethics consultant, to include a self-assessment form, a record of all relevant education and training, a record of consultations performed, and a summary of evaluations from the consultations.

Conclusion

Improving quality in ethics consultations requires enhancing the accountability of individual ethics consultants and ethics committees. First, consultants and committees need to do some self-assessment. Second, they must seek out educational programs and opportunities to link with ethics centers, networks, or other resources to work together to explore challenging ethical issues and to enhance the functioning of ethics consultation mechanisms. Finally, and equally important, consultants' performance should be evaluated every step of the way, from entire ethics programs to individual consultations and consultants. Without actively participating in a well-organized and comprehensive ethics education program, ethics consultants may lack the necessary core competencies to ensure quality in the consultation process.

Acknowledgments

The authors acknowledge and thank the following people, who provided helpful information about their programs: Barbara L. Chanko, R.N., M.B.A.; Kenneth A. Berkowitz, M.D.; Mark P. Aulisio, Ph.D.; Janet Fleetwood, Ph.D.; Jack Glaser, Ph.D.; Elaine Glass, R.N., M.S.; Mark Kuczewski, Ph.D.; Sue Rubin, Ph.D.; and Tom Tomlinson, Ph.D.

Disclaimer

The views expressed in this chapter by William Nelson are his alone and do not represent the views of the Department of Veterans Affairs or the U.S. government.

Notes

1. Fletcher, J.C., "Standards for Evaluation of Ethics Consultation," in *Ethics Consultation in Health Care,* ed. J.C. Fletcher, N. Quist, and A.R.E. Jonsen (Ann Arbor, Mich.: Health Administration Press, 1989), pp. 173-84.

2. Aulisio, M.P., Arnold, R.M., and Youngner, S.J., "Can There Be Educational and Training Standards for Those Conducting Health Care Ethics Consultations?" in *Health Care Ethics: Critical Issues for the Twenty-First Century,* ed. D. Thomasma and J. Monagle (Gaithersburg, Md.: Aspen Press, 1998), pp. 484–96; Baylis, F.E., "A Profile of the Health Care Ethics Consultant," in *The Health Care Ethics Consultant,* ed. F. Baylis (Totowa, N.J.: Humana Press, 1994), pp. 89–99; Fletcher, J.C., Quist, N., and Jonsen, A.R.E., eds., *Ethics Consultation in Health Care* (Ann Arbor, Mich.: Health Administration Press, 1989); Fletcher, J.C., and Hoffman, D.E., "Ethics Committees: Time to Experiment with Standards," *Annals of Internal Medicine* 120 (1994):335- 37; Fleetwood, J., and Unger, S.S., "Institutional Ethics Committees and the Shield of Immunity," *Annals of Internal Medicine* 120 (1994):320–25; LaPuma, J., and Toulmin, S.E., "Ethics Consultants and Ethics Committees," *Annals of Internal Medicine* 149 (1989):1109–12.

3. Society for Health and Human Values–Society for Bioethics Consultation: Task Force on Standards for Bioethics Consultation, *Core Competencies for Health Care Ethics Consultation: The Report of the American Society for Bioethics and Humanities* (Glenview, Ill.: American Society for Bioethics and Humanities, 1998).

4. Nelson, W., and Wlody, G., "The Evolving Role of Ethics Advisory Committees in VHA," *HEC Forum* 9 (1997):129–46.

5. ASBH report, p. 11.

6. Davis, D., O'Brian, M.A., Freemantle, N., Wolf, F.M., Mazmanian, P., and Taylor-

Vaisey, A., "Impact of Formal Continuing Education," *Journal of the American Medical Association* 120 (1999):867–74.

7. Moss, A.H., "The Application of the Task Force Report in Rural and Frontier Settings," *Journal of Clinical Ethics* 10, no. 1 (1999):42–48.

8. Nelson, W., and Law, D., "Clinical Ethics Education in the Department of Veterans Affairs," *Cambridge Quarterly of Healthcare Ethics* 3, no. 1 (1994):142–48.

9. Davis et al., "Impact of Formal Continuing Education."

10. American Society for Bioethics and Humanities, *North American Graduate Bioethics and Medical Humanities Training Program Survey* (Glenview, Ill.: ASBH Status of the Field Committee, October 2001).

11. Fox, E., "Concepts in Evaluation Applied to Ethics Consultant Research," *Journal of Clinical Ethics* 7, no. 2 (1996):116–21; Fox, E., and Arnold, R.M., "Evaluating Outcomes in Ethics Consultation Research," *Journal of Clinical Ethics* 7, no. 2 (1996):127–38; Fox, E., and Tulsky, J., "Evaluation Research and the Future of Ethics Consultation," *Journal of Clinical Ethics* 7, no. 2 (1996):146–49; Tulsky, J., and Fox, E., "Evaluating Ethics Consultations: Framing the Questions," *Journal of Clinical Ethics* 7, no. 2 (1996):139–45.

12. Orr, R.D., "Evaluation of an Ethics Consultation Service: Patient and Family Perspective," *American Journal of Medicine* 101 (1996):135–41.

5

Techniques for Training Ethics Consultants:

Why Traditional Classroom Methods Are Not Enough

ROBERT M. ARNOLD, M.D., AND

MELANIE H. WILSON SILVER, PH.D.

Imagine that your 15-year-old daughter says she wants to learn to play the violin. To help her, you begin by looking into the available music courses in your community, only to find that most programs consist of ninety hours of music theory, five hours of watching an expert violinist play, and five hours of practice time. You will probably conclude that these programs are inadequate to teach your daughter to play the violin.

The purpose of this chapter is to suggest that a similar (or worse) prospect faces most people who wish to learn to participate in ethics consultations. First, we briefly review some common conceptions about the ethics consultant's role and the tasks needed to fulfill this role. Then we review the meager empirical literature on the training of ethics consultants and argue that consultants are undertrained, particularly in facilitation. We conclude that, if one believes the recommendations of the Task Force on Standards for Bioethics Consultation, most individuals are poorly trained to perform consultations. Finally, we attempt to apply Daniel Schon's theory of reflective practice to ethics consultation and argue that training requires more attention to daily practice.[1] This means that consultants-in-training should be directly observed and provided with feedback about their decision making.

First, however, some cautionary notes. As noted above, the information on how ethics consultants actually are trained is meager. The data that do exist are fragmentary and describe consultants' academic backgrounds rather than their educational experiences. Thus, our comments on training are impressionistic and based on our experiences and discussions with colleagues. Second, we also lack data on consultants' current knowledge and skills, and rather than making the more convincing claim that lack of skill-based education results in decreased competency, the best we can do is to reference data from other fields. Third, the chapter's major point, that training should focus more on the skills and knowledge needed for ethics facilitation, is not meant to denigrate ethical theory and its importance in clinical decision making. Rather, we wish to underscore what we see as a current deficiency in the training of consultants. Fourth, the chapter speaks of an "ethics consultant." We use this term for convenience only, not because we think consultations are better performed by a single individual than by a group or committee. We believe the arguments presented here have the same force when applied to individuals or groups performing consultations. Finally, this chapter focuses solely on the training needed for ethics consultation, which is not the same as the training needed to teach ethics (to medical students, residents, health professionals, bioethics students, or any other relevant group), to perform policy analysis, or for any other tasks.

Conceptions of Bioethics Consultation

The ASBH task force defined health care ethics consultation as "a service provided by an individual or group to help patients, families, surrogates, health care providers, or other involved parties address uncertainty or conflict regarding value-laden issues that emerge in health care." The task force conceptualized the ethics consultants' role to be that of an "ethics facilitator." Rather than imposing the *consultant's* view of what would be morally correct, the ethics consultant works with the patient, family, and health care provider to facilitate a decision that is consistent with *their* values. The boundaries of the consensus are set not by the consultant's values but by "societal values, law, and institutional policy." To accomplish this task, consultants must "gather relevant data, clarify relevant concepts, clarify related normative issues and help to identify a range of morally acceptable options within the context."[2]

Others have suggested similar roles for ethics consultants. Casarett and Daskal apply Habermas's theory of discourse ethics to provide a basis for a model of consultation grounded in consensus and communication. They describe the consultant as a "facilitator" who "sets the stage and arranges the props to facilitate moral argumentation. As a facilitator, their role is hermeneutic, conciliatory, and directed toward the establishment of a dialogue that can lead to consensus." They speak of "gathering data, enhancing communication, identifying areas of ethical discomfort, and clarifying the goals of participants" as core functions of a consultant.[3] Walker describes consultants as architects and mediators. As architects, they work to keep open a moral space in which all parties can state their views within the constraints of the particular institution. As mediators, they "actively participate in a situation with a primary commitment to a fruitful process of resolution."[4] Finally, Orr and deLeon speak of consultants serving as conflict mediators—as negotiators, mediators, and arbitrators.[5]

A recent empirical study supports this role for ethics consultants. Jurchack surveyed the members of the Society for Bioethics Consultation on the frequency with which they participated in certain tasks. She found that consultants frequently engage in behaviors consistent with ethics facilitation: "gathering facts, identifying moral principles, ensuring inclusiveness of all involved parties in discussion, exploring mutual perspectives, identifying common points of interest, facilitating mutual respect among parties, joint problem solving."[6] The vast majority of ethics consultations are the result of communication difficulties—ranging from a lack of communication to miscommunication or mistaken beliefs about what the law, hospital policy, or clinical medicine requires.[7] The cases that raise ethically difficult situations (e.g., difficulty in identifying an appropriate decision maker and/or an appropriate decision) are much less common.[8]

Competencies Required to Serve as an Ethics Facilitator

The task force attempted to describe the knowledge and skills needed both for ethical analysis and for facilitating a consensus. The requirements for knowledge of ethical theory are not controversial. Consultants must have a knowledge of ethical theory generally and bioethics more specifically. They must have a familiarity with both societal laws and the hospital's policies. Casarett and Daskal summarize the importance of knowing ethical theory: "The goal of consultation should be an understanding of the roots of the disagreement and of the path toward resolution. An understanding of moral theory is essential toward this task."[9] The task force also noted that knowledge of ethical theory is required to help delineate the boundary conditions within which the case operates and determine what should be done should a consensus not be reached.

The task force also concluded that a consultant needs certain analytical skills to illuminate the ethical issues surrounding a consultation. She must be able to identify the nature of the value uncertainty or conflict that underlies the need for consultation. Ethical issues must be distinguished from other, social and interpersonal issues for which a social worker or psychiatrist may be more appropriate. Having done this, the consultant must be able to analyze the participants' views, help them see the different values that underlie their decision making, and help them identify morally acceptable options. This requires the ability to identify, clarify, and critically evaluate relevant ethical and bio-ethical concepts.

Besides the knowledge and skills needed to deal with the ethical aspects of the case, equally important are the knowledge and skills needed to serve as a competent facilitator.[10] These competencies were not discussed in the early literature on ethics consultation. However, the ASBH report emphasizes the role of facilitation and the skills one needs to accomplish this task: the abilities to set ground rules for formal meetings, to create an atmosphere of trust, to negotiate between competing moral views, and to do creative problem solving. The report also emphasizes the importance of interpersonal skills such as listening well; communicating interest, respect, support, and empathy; and being able to represent the views of the involved parties to each other.

It is interesting, however, that the task force had little to say about the *knowledge* required to facilitate conflict resolution. There is a large body of knowledge on conflict-based mediation, both narrowly focused within medical ethics and more generally covered in the business literature,[11] that discusses how people make decisions, the common reasons why conflicts occur, their cognitive and emotional causes, and their relative frequency. The literature also describes various methods for structuring conflict resolution and their success in different situations.

We believe that basic knowledge about group process, mediation, and conflict resolution should be part of ethics consultants' training. It would not be enough for surgeons to have the ability to competently cut or sew, without a knowledge of the anatomical structures on which they are operating. Similarly, ethics consultants require more than just the facilitative skills needed to be a competent facilitator. They must have an understanding of the process by which conflicts arise and are resolved. Moreover, in order to create a safe environment for the discussion of ethical issues, ethics facilitators need to understand how the power differential among health care providers can influence conversations. Consultants also need to understand concepts such as active listening, mirroring, brainstorming, and premature closure, and the relevance of these concepts to group process and decision making.

Training for an Ethics Facilitator

The literature on training for health care ethics consultants has focused on ensuring adequate knowledge about bioethics and the ability to analyze ethical issues (see Chapter 4). The reasons for this are relatively straightforward. First, the older literature on ethics consultation emphasized the theoretical aspects of cases and the importance of ethical theory in their resolution. Learning the principles of bioethics and how to apply them to clinical cases was thus seen as central to consultation. Later in the evolution of bioethics, when other methodologies became popular, the emphasis stayed on theoretical concerns. Thus, for example, consultants learning casuistry emphasized the importance of identifying paradigmatic cases, clarifying the variables that differentiated cases, and learning to place the case in question within this schema. Second, the paradigmatic cases that were used to train consultants focused on such ethical issues as decision-making capacity, confidentiality, or foregoing life-sustaining treatment. Thus it seemed that the best tool to "solve" the case was ethical theory. Third, ethical theory was, in part, what distinguished ethics consultation from other types of consultation in health care settings. Conflicts in hospitals were often mediated by social workers, patients' representatives, administrators, or lawyers. However, in the 1970s there was a call for "ethics" committees and consultants to become involved in dealing with disputes about end-of-life care. The key factor that differentiated these consultants from others who might help resolve conflict was their knowledge of ethical theory. This also justified the role of philosophers in the medical center. Not surprisingly, then, for philosophers and theologians, what differentiated them from others was what was crucial about ethics consultation. Finally, ethical theory was the topic least likely to be taught to health care providers who wanted to be hospital ethics consultants. Health care providers did not receive much training in bioethics, so this was an area of perceived need.

Given these factors, the emphasis on ensuring adequate training in bioethical concepts and associated analytical skills is understandable. A number of different programs developed to fill this need. Ethics committees set up self-directed reading groups, often led by a philosopher or theologian with expertise in ethical theory. These groups read articles on ethical theories and bioethical concepts and discussed their importance and relevance to clinical situations. The groups often referred to paradigmatic case scenarios in the literature to discuss how the different theories and concepts could be applied to "resolving" the conflict. (More recently, the discussion has emphasized the role of different theoretical constructs to ethical conflicts.)

Conferences offer opportunities to obtain similar knowledge and skills in a more concentrated manner. Many academic ethics centers offer one- to two-week meetings in basic or advanced topics in bioethics. These conferences cover, in a survey fashion, the most common issues confronting ethics consultants in a hospital setting. The conference typically consists of a combination of lecture and small-group case-based discussions. A number of these programs give certificates in bioethics at the completion of the sessions.

Finally, for individuals who want a more advanced background in bioethical concepts and analytical skills, some universities offer an M.A. or Ph.D. degree or a Doctorate in Health Care Ethics. These programs require students to take a number of in-depth courses covering both ethical theory and common bioethical concepts. Many of the programs are more appropriate for full-time consultants or educators and scholars in bioethics than for those working part-time in ethics consultation.

Hoffman and colleagues recently surveyed 466 ethics committee members in Maryland who performed consultations, and inquired about their education in ethical theory. Of the consultants surveyed, 192 (41 percent) responded. Seventy-three had some formal education in bioethics—two had master's degrees, twenty-two had a certificate from a bioethics program, twenty-eight had a Ph.D. or master's degree in ethics, and twenty-one had a B.A. in philosophy or religious studies. While most did not have formal degrees or certificates in bioethics, respondents reported attending, on average, 4.3 hours of in-service education relevant to ethics consultation in 1998 and 5.4 hours of out-of-hospital education. Interestingly, 30 percent of consultants said they received zero hours of either in-service or out-of-hospital education in 1997. Individuals who had performed consultations in 1997 were more likely to have attended educational programs related to consultation. Hoffman and colleagues found a statistical correlation between respondents' perceived competency in ethics assessment skills and formal training in ethics, but the differences were small.[12]

The results of this survey are cause for concern. Despite the literature and the numerous programs focusing on the importance of bioethical theory and concepts to ethics consultation, the survey results suggest that more than half of individuals performing ethics consultation in Maryland have no formal education in ethics or bioethical analysis. One hopes that these individuals are performing consultations only with colleagues who have had training. Moreover, to ensure at least minimal competency one would expect consultants to have some continuing education in ethics. But 30 percent of consultants responding to the survey did not attend any educational programs in 1997.

Attending courses is obviously not enough—competency is what concerned the task force most. The degree to which these courses accomplish their purpose is unknown. There is no empirical research examining the effect of such courses on ethics consultants' knowledge of ethical theory or their analytical skills. Some data are available on the effectiveness of teaching medical ethics to medical students and house officers; they suggest that medical ethics education may improve students' moral reasoning and ability to identify ethical issues. The data on whether such training affects students' actual behavior are much more controversial.[13] However, some research has looked at the relative efficacy of different educational techniques for accomplishing certain goals. For example, recent research has shown that a time-honored method of teaching doctors—lectures in large auditoriums—is not the best way of improving their knowledge. Thus, insofar as the courses outlined above are designed to ensure knowledge of bioethical concepts or analytical skills, educational interventions for consultants should be structured along the following principles:

- *Adult learners are problem-centered* and relate new learning to prior experiences. They are stimulated by problem-centered rather than subject-centered approaches to learning.[14] Thus, learning experiences should focus on helping individuals develop competence in mastering tasks that they consider important and difficult.

- *Experiential education is more likely to change behavior* than are didactic interventions. For example, lectures are less likely than seminar discussions to lead to improved analytical skills.

- *Small-group-based education is an effective educational technique,* as effective as individual study, if not more so. Groups can facilitate the learning process by allowing participants to share what they know, rather than assuming that the teacher is the sole fund of knowledge on which learners can draw.[15] Thus Self found that teaching medical ethics through case discussions in small groups was more likely than large-group discussions to improve students' moral reasoning.[16]

- *Practice is essential for acquiring skills.* The process of learning new skills is best taught by actually practicing new behaviors rather than just reading or hearing about them. Also, research shows that learning is enhanced if the behaviors are taught over multiple sessions rather than lumped into one session.[17] Feedback, as close to the time of the practiced behavior as possible, is an important part of the learning process.[18]

- *Modeling helps learners understand and acquire behavior,* better than does listening to a talk. Vicarious modeling—observing and critiquing others' behavior—and participant modeling are important to the learning process.[19]

The degree to which current educational interventions for ethics consultants incorporate these pedagogical techniques is unknown. We can conclude, however, that different kinds of courses are needed to ensure different competencies:

• Didactic sessions and readings may be useful for teaching consultants about basic competencies in a time-efficient manner.

• More interactive sessions, such as graduate seminars and case-based discussions, can help consultants understand concepts and their role in decision making. These sessions may also help consultants learn how best to inquire about another person's beliefs (although this would require discussion in a less confrontational manner than sometimes occurs in traditional philosophy courses).

• Educational interventions that require participants to work through individual cases and then justify their answers in small groups can improve analytical skills and help participants apply concepts in "real-life" situations. These interventions also provide a forum for learning about small-group process and negotiation.

In recent years there has been a growth in distance learning and self-directed educational opportunities in medical ethics. These courses offer a flexible way for individuals to obtain training in medical ethics and may be particularly useful in locales with limited access to ethics education. Moreover, readings (either alone or in a small group) are a wonderful way to learn much of the cognitive material discussed in this chapter. Group discussions can allow individuals to begin practicing the analytical skills needed to help individuals resolve difficult cases. However, self-directed learning has limitations. In isolation, it cannot prepare students to achieve the optimal or necessary level of interactive experience or expose them to opportunities to learn and improve communication skills. Self-education alone is unlikely to teach the skills necessary to becoming a competent facilitator; this requires an interactive and modeling component as part of the educational process. Distance learning could overcome these barriers by using interactive videos and computers, but we are not aware of any programs that currently have this focus.

Teaching Facilitation: Knowledge and Skills

A larger problem is the lack of education on group process, decision making, and facilitation. What few empirical data exist suggest that underlying the call for most ethics consultations is either a lack of communication or a miscommunication rather than a complex ethical issue. In our personal experience this is clearly the case. Knowledge of how individuals make decisions when under stress, common etiologies for miscommunication, and conflict-resolution techniques are likely to be more helpful in resolving interpersonal conflicts than knowledge about various formulations of the categorical imperative.

Nevertheless, few programs deal with this body of knowledge in the training of ethics consultants. We know of only one short course on ethics consultation that deals explicitly with mediation techniques (a certification program offered by N. Dubler at Montefiore Medical Center). Few ethics committees include materials on facilitation or group process among their core readings. Only at the master's degree and Ph.D. program level are these topics covered in a systematic manner (and even here, only a minority of programs require such a course).

A variety of reasons underlie the lack of explicit instruction on mediation. First, some may believe there is no body of knowledge to teach. Critics argue that improving communication between individuals is a basic human skill that a person does or does not have. We cannot teach individuals to be facilitative. The intellectual basis is a matter of common sense. There is nothing to learn. In fact, there is a large body of theoretical and empirical information that disproves this objection. Data from a number of disciplines, including psychology, sociology, communication studies, and business, have shown that

- certain groups go through certain typical phases that influence their effective functioning;
- "normal" conversations lead to errors in understanding and may reinforce power differentials;
- interpersonal decision making is influenced by a variety of environmental and situational factors;
- under stress, individuals' decision making is prone to certain common logical errors;
- biases influence decision making; and
- certain interpersonal techniques are likely to help individuals achieve consensus in difficult decisions.[20]

Moreover, many psychology, law, and business schools have courses focusing on group decision making, negotiation, and/or mediation. These programs have texts and professors with academic careers in research on decision making, group process, facilitation, and negotiation, all of which suggest there is a body of knowledge to be learned.

Second, some may believe that instruction in mediation techniques is ethically questionable. Acquiring these skills, critics argue, raises the specter of slick consultants convincing less-skilled parties to agreements they would otherwise oppose. Popular books and courses, such as the Karras training courses on negotiation, may reinforce the idea that these are manipulative methods by which some can accomplish their goals at the expense of others. What should count in ethics consultation is the *ethical* aspects of the case, not how "good" the consultant is at facilitation.

It is true that interpersonal techniques may be used for illicit purposes. One could imagine, à la the unscrupulous used-car salesperson, a group of ethics consultants "convincing" a family to forgo life-sustaining treatment for their loved one. However, this would be a misuse of mediation skills. The goal of mediation is to help the involved parties come to a mutually agreeable decision, not to convince them to do what you think should be done. Moreover, we need to remember that the role of consultation is *ethics* facilitation. The facilitative knowledge and skills are not to be valued in and of themselves. The skills are to be used to promote an ethically justifiable consensus—a consensus that reflects the values of the involved parties and is located within the societal consensus. The facilitative skills are to be used to ensure that all parties' voices are heard, to help clear up misunderstandings, and to help "discover" common grounds for deliberation. To use Walker's language, ethics consultants use facilitation to "keep moral spaces open," to "foster and nurture a collective and collaborative moral process."[21]

Third, some may believe that such knowledge is important but that specific training is redundant. Health care providers have already acquired basic knowledge in these areas in school, rendering this additional learning extraneous for ethics consultation. To our knowledge this is not the case. No medical school explicitly deals with these topics. In fact, most provide little training in communication skills after the first year of medical school.[22] A good deal of information documents the limitations of physicians' communication skills. While nursing schools and social workers' programs do spend more time teaching communication skills, many do not have explicit training in negotiation. The goal of health care providers is typically to convince others to modify their behavior in certain ways, not to encourage deeper understanding or to negotiate a joint agreement. Finally, most philosophy Ph.D. programs do not include training in these areas. As recent books on bioethics emphasize, determining truth has a longer pedigree in philosophy than does attempting to promote consensus.[23] Moreover, the training in teaching skills, communication, or group process is often scanty in graduate school.

Finally, critics may argue that knowledge about mediation is extraneous because what counts is "negotiation skills" rather than knowledge about negotiation. Facilitation is an activity rather than a knowledge set. One may know and be able to describe the interpersonal factors that promote consensus, but be unable to carry out these tasks.

There is some truth to this objection. Ethics consultation is an interpersonal activity. We should be much more interested in facilitative skills than in knowledge about facilitation. This is probably why the task force deemphasized knowledge about facilitation in the list of competencies. Still, we should be careful in how far we push this argument. For many individuals, knowledge does improve action. Knowing the best way to organize a meeting, for example, makes it more likely that someone will act to organize a meeting in this manner. Knowing the most common misunderstandings in group deliberations, a facilitator is more likely to inquire about these misunderstandings. Knowledge is not important for its own sake, but there is reason to think that knowledge about facilitation will improve facilitation skills.

This last objection is correct in emphasizing the primacy of facilitation skills. The problem is that the lack of training in such skills is striking among most consultants. Most programs of which we are aware provide no formal training on the ability to:

- listen well and to communicate interest, respect, support, and empathy to involved parties
- educate involved parties regarding the ethical dimensions of the case
- elicit the moral views of involved parties
- represent the views of involved parties to others
- enable involved parties to communicate effectively and be heard by other parties
- recognize and attend to various relational barriers to communication.[24]

These abilities can be taught through informal role modeling. For example, some programs require that less-experienced consultants "shadow" more experienced ones and observe the process of consultation. More rarely do programs have senior consultants watch junior ones "do" consultations and give them feedback on their communication skills. Even when this occurs, learning may be minimal. The problem is that unless the senior consultants have insight into the process of negotiation, they are unlikely to be able to highlight the important steps for the junior consultant. The junior consultant, who also lacks any knowledge about mediation, may be unable to understand why one consultant seems "better" than another. The resulting training, if it occurs at all, will be slow and characterized largely by trial and error.

In our experience, even this informal education rarely occurs. The importance of process in ethics consultation is underappreciated. While consultants ask about whether certain data have been collected (and their relevance to decision making), they generally ignore how the information is collected and its importance to the consultation.

This problem is magnified because these skills are not adequately taught in consultants' primary discipline. Social workers may well have had some training in these areas—particularly if they took courses in group counseling. Similarly, hospital chaplains, depending on their training, may have practiced these skills. But although most medical schools provide some training in communication skills, it is relatively meager and focused in the preclinical years. Moreover, data suggesting that doctors typically interrupt a patient after less than twenty seconds do not increase one's confidence in their facilitative skills. (And in our experience, lack of adequate communication with the health care provider is the etiology of many ethics consultations.) Those who come to consultation from philosophy, religious studies, or law also are unlikely to have much formal training in facilitative techniques. And, though some of the techniques are the same as might be used in the business world, their application in the emotionally stressful hospital setting is different. Complicating matters is the fact that most consultation is done by groups of consultants. Ideally, the consultants would have some training in co-facilitation, something we have never seen.

These skills could be taught in a number of ways. The focus has to be on practice, feedback, and more practice. To quote from the ASBH report:

Process and interpersonal skills are acquired primarily by "doing." There is no substitute for the role of experience in their development. One may be able to discuss how to facilitate a formal meeting, for example, but until one actually gains experience in facilitating formal meetings, one will not adequately develop the skill. Basic interpersonal and process skills should be engendered through educational and training opportunities that are interactive and experientially based. Presentations and in-service sessions at one's local institution which include role-playing a case consultation, or running a simulated meeting would be good ways to begin to acquire basic process and interpersonal skills. Short intensive courses focused on developing these skills should also be adequate. Course work in interpersonal communication, psychology, sociology, education, or social work, provided that it includes significant interactive components, should engender basic skill in these areas as well.[25]

The teaching of psychotherapy skills is an instructive example (although the requirements are much lower for ethics consultation). As in ethics consultation, learning to "do" psychotherapy requires a theoretical basis (and as in bioethics, there is no agreement on the "correct" theory). Regardless, most programs require a large amount of observed practice (often after watching a trained practitioner). Techniques used to accomplish this include standardized patients, audiotaping and videotaping, and personal observation of consultations. Similar training could be required for ethics consultants.

One might object that this material (like knowledge about mediation) cannot be taught. One either is or is not a good facilitator, critics would say. These skills are developed early in human development, and courses taken in adulthood are unlikely to make a difference. This objection may have some truth to it. It is unlikely that a few courses in facilitation will make major changes in someone's communication skills. Certain types of individuals are probably unsuited to consultation. For example, individuals with a highly authoritarian style will probably retain this style after training as an ethics consultant and probably are ill suited for the task. However, many individuals could become consultants but are unsure how to facilitate a meeting or mediate disagreements. These individuals lack specific skills. Data increasingly suggest that interactive courses in communication can improve health care providers' communication skills.[26] It is likely that similar courses could improve consultants' ability to perform ethics facilitation.

Praxis

Daniel Schon's work on educating the reflective practitioner may provide a better sense of the importance of "hands-on" training for ethics consultation.[27] Schon argues that professions such as medicine, engineering, and law are characterized by the artistry and reflection in action ("the 'thinking what they are doing while they are doing it'") that practitioners bring to situations of uncertainty, uniqueness, and conflict. (This argument works regardless of whether one thinks ethics consultation is a "profession.") These skills are "an exercise of intelligence, a kind of knowing . . . [The artistry] is not inherently mysterious; it is rigorous in its own terms."[28] The artistry of the practice is required to frame the problem, implement interventions, and improvise when faced with novel situations. The artistry consists of learning to think like a doctor, lawyer, or engineer. This process helps the practitioner deal with indeterminate situations in which there is "no obvious fit between the characteristics of the situation and the available body of theories and techniques" (p. 6). In these situations, a practitioner responds to the unexpected by "restructuring some of her strategies of action, theories of the phenomena or ways of framing the problem; and she invents on the spot experiments to put her new understandings to the test" (p. 38). For example, a doctor seeing a patient with an unusual set of symptoms will rethink the traditional diagnostic categories and then test the new differential.

Unfortunately, Schon argues, traditional education focuses on teaching technical rationality that "holds that practitioners are instrumental problem solvers who select technical means best suited to particular purposes (p. 10). Doctors thus work by applying systematic, scientific knowledge to well-formed problems. This framework of education, however, has failed to realize the degree to which real-world practice presents itself not as clearly defined problems but as "messy, indeterminate situations." "If they [doctors] are to get to a well-formed problem matched to their familiar theories and techniques, they must *construct* it from the material of a situation" (p. 10). Learning to do this requires artistry, not technical rationality.

Artistry is taught through practice. Schon's paradigmatic example is a practicum. "In a setting that approximates a practice world, students learn by doing, although their work usually falls short of real-world work" (p. 37). In the practicum, the student must learn the fundamental tasks of competent practice. "She must learn the 'practice of the practicum'—its tools, methods, projects and possibilities—and assimilate to it her emerging image of how she can best learn what she wants to learn" (p. 37).

This work is accomplished by both reflecting on what one is doing and being coached by a teacher. The coaching will take many forms—ranging from demonstrating to advising, questioning, and criticizing. The goal is to help practitioners "recognize and apply standard rules, facts and operations; then to reason from general rules to problematic cases in ways characteristic of the profession; and . . . to develop and test new forms of understanding and action where familiar categories and ways of thinking fail" (p. 39). (Schon's interest and emphasis is largely with the third of these tasks.)

What is the relevance of this to ethics consultation? First, we believe the task of ethics consultation is a practice, like medicine and engineering, in which artistry is a central component. In both facilitating and analyzing the ethical problem, consultants must learn to reflect on what they are doing while they act and must learn to "work outside the box," attempting new ways of working with people in crisis. Particularly in medical ethics, given the rapid advances in technologies and growing cultural diversity, consultants must test new "categories of understanding, strategies of action and ways of framing problems" (p. 38). Second, if this is accurate, then the training of consultants must allow for both application of applied knowledge (bioethics and facilitation) and coaching in the artistry of reflection in action (ethical analysis, problem solving, and facilitation). Third, this means that the training of ethics consultants requires opportunities for practicums in which students can both observe and be observed. This could be done in a number of different ways—direct observation, developing "mock ethics cases" with other students or standardized patients, audiotaping consultations for review, or requiring extended commentaries and debriefing.[29] Finally, the instruction of consultants will need to be revamped, with less emphasis on theory and more on how a consultant thinks through a case. This "reflection in action" requires participants to reflect aloud on their decision making—why they chose to talk to this person rather than that person, why they asked about the patient's values, what ethical considerations they were thinking about, and so forth. Others then comment on these reflections in an attempt to help students understand the process of "expert" consultation.

Conclusion

The task force argued that the role of the ethics consultant is to facilitate ethically and that this requires certain competencies. We agree with these underlying assumptions. The purpose of this chapter has been to point out their educational implications. We believe education of the ethics consultant needs to focus more attention on the facilitative aspects of a consultant's job. This, in turn, requires a transition from the classroom to the practicum. Performance should be as important as, if not more important than, talking about the issues. Otherwise one runs the risk that the training of ethics consultants, like the teaching of the violinist in the introductory story, will be "all talk and no show."

Notes

1. Schon, D., *Educating the Reflective Practitioner* (San Francisco: Jossey-Bass, 1987).

2. Society for Health and Human Values–Society for Bioethics Consultation: Task Force on Standards for Bioethics Consultation, *Core Competencies for Health Care Ethics Consultation: The Report of the American Society for Bioethics and Humanities* (Glenview, Ill.: American Society for Bioethics and Humanities, 1998), p. 6.

3. Casarett, D.J, and Daskal, F., "The Authority of the Clinical Ethicist," *Hastings Center Report* 28 (1998):6–10, see p. 8.

4. Walker, M.U., "Keeping Moral Spaces Open: New Images of Ethics Consulting," *Hastings Center Report* 23 (1993):33–40, see p. 40.

5. Orr, R.D., and deLeon, D.M., "The Role of the Clinical Ethicist in Conflict Resolution," *Journal of Clinical Ethics* 11 (2000):21–30.

6. Jurchack, M., "Report of a Study to Examine the Process of Ethics Case Consultation," *Journal of Clinical Ethics* 11 (2000):49–55.

7. DuVal, G., Sartorius, L., Clarridge, B., Gensler, G., and Danis, M., "What Triggers Requests for Ethics Consultations?" *Western Journal of Medicine* 175 (2001):24–30.

8. La Puma, J., "Consultations in Clinical Ethics—Issues and Questions in 27 Cases," *Western Journal of Medicine* 146 (1987):633–37; La Puma, J., Stocking, C.B., Silverstein, M.D., DiMartini, D., and Siegler, M., "An Ethics Consultation Service in a Teaching Hospital: Utilization and Evaluation," *Journal of the American Medical Association* 260 (1988):808–11.

9. Casarett and Daskal, "Authority of the Clinical Ethicist."

10. West, M.B., and Gibson, J.M., "Facilitating Medical Ethics Case Review: What Ethics Committees Can Learn from Mediation and Facilitation Techniques," *Cambridge Quarterly of Healthcare Ethics* 1, no. 1 (1992):63–74; Orr and deLeon, "Role of the Clinical Ethicist"; Dubler, N., and Libman, C.B., *Mediating Bioethical Disputes: Seeking Consensus among Conflicting Interests* (New York: United Hospital Fund, 2001).

11. Hunter, D., and Bailey, A., *The Art of Facilitation: How to Create Group Synergy* (Tucson, Ariz.: Fisher Books, 1995); Ackerman, T.F., "Conceptualizing the Role of the Ethics Consultant: Some Theoretical Issues," in *Ethics Consultation in Health Care,* ed. J.C. Fletcher, N. Quist, and A.R.E. Jonsen (Ann Arbor, Mich.: Health Administration Press, 1989), pp. 37–52; Fleetwood, J.E., Arnold, R.M., and Baron, R.J., "Giving Answers or Raising Questions? The Problematic Role of Institutional Ethics Committees," *Journal of Medical Ethics* 15 (1989):137–42; Neale, M., *Cognition and Rationality in Negotiation* (New York: Free Press, 1991); West, M.B., "Mediation and Communication Techniques in Ethics Consultation," *Journal of Clinical Ethics* 3 (1992):291–92; West, M.B., and Gibson, J.M., "Facilitating Medical Ethics Case Review: What Ethics Committees Can Learn from Mediation and Facilitation Techniques," *Cambridge Quarterly of Healthcare Ethics* 1 (1992):63–74; Agich, G.J., "Expertise in Clinical Ethics Consultation," *HEC Forum* 6 (1994):379–83; Baylis, F.E., "A Profile of the Health Care Ethics Consultant," in *The Health Care Ethics Consultant,* ed. F.E. Baylis (Totowa, N.J.: Humana Press, 1994), pp. 25–

44; Gibson, K., "Biases and Rationality in the Mediation Process," in *Applications of Heuristics and Biases to Social Issues* (New York: Plenum Press, 1994); Lynch, A., ". . . Has Knowledge of [Interpersonal] Facilitation Techniques and Theory; Has the Ability to Facilitate [Interpersonally] . . . : Fact or Fiction?" in Bayliss, *Health Care Ethics Consultant*, pp. 45–62; Schwarz, R., *The Skilled Facilitator* (San Francisco: Jossey-Bass, 1994); Crigger, B., "Negotiating the Moral Order: Paradoxes of Ethics Consultation," *Kennedy Institute of Ethics Journal* 5 (1995):89–112; Gibson, K., "Mediation in the Medical Field: Is Neutral Intervention Possible?" *Hastings Center Report* 29 (1999):6–13.

12. Hoffman, D., Tarzian, A., and O'Neil, A., "Are Ethics Committee Members Competent to Consult?" *Journal of Law, Medicine and Ethics* 28 (2000):30–40.

13. Fox E., Arnold R.M., and Brody B., "Medical Ethics Education: Past, Present and Future," *Academic Medicine* 70 (1995):761–69; Arnold, R.M., and Forrow, B.L., "Assessing Compliance in Clinical Ethics: Are We Measuring the Right Behaviors?" *Journal of General Internal Medicine* 8 (1993):52–54.

14. Knowles, M.S., *The Modern Practice of Adult Education* (New York: State University of New York Press, 1996); Knowles, M.S., *The Modern Practice of Adult Education: From Pedagogy to Androgyny* (New York: Globe Fearon Educational Publishing, 1988).

15. Cartwright, D., and Zander, A., *Group Dynamics: Research and Theory* (Evanston, Ill.: Row, Peterson and Co., 1953); Lipkin, M., Putnam, S.M., and Lazare, A., eds., *The Medical Interview: Clinical Care, Education, and Research* (New York: Springer Publishing, 1995).

16. Self, D.J., "The Educational Philosophies behind the Medical Humanities Programs in the United States: An Empirical Assessment of Three Different Approaches to Humanistic Medical Education," *Theoretical Medicine* 14, no. 3 (1993):221–29.

17. Maguire, P., and Faulkner, A., "Improve the Counseling Skills of Doctors and Nurses in Cancer Care," *British Medical Journal* 297 (1998):847-49.

18. Ende, J., "Feedback in Clinical Medical Education," *Journal of the American Medical Association* 250 (1983):777–81; Skeff, K.M., Berman, J., and Stratos, G., *A Review of Clinical Teaching Improvement Methods and a Theoretical Framework for Their Evaluation* (New York: Springer Publishing, 1988).

19. Rosenthal, T., and Bandura, A., "Psychological Modeling: Theory and Practice," in *Handbook of Psychotherapy and Behavior Change: An Empirical Analysis*, ed. S. Garfield and A. Bergin (New York: Wiley, 1978); Skeff, K.M., and Mutha, S., "Role Models: Guiding the Future of Medicine" (editorial), *New England Journal of Medicine* 339, no. 27 (1987):2015–17.

20. Hunter and Bailey, *The Art of Facilitation;* Huckaby and Neuman, *Managing Cofacilitation;* Ackerman, "Conceptualizing the Role of the Ethics Consultant"; Fleetwood et al., "Giving Answers or Raising Questions?"; Neale, *Cognition and Rationality in Negotiation;* West, "Mediation and Communication Techniques"; West and Gibson, "Facilitating Medical Ethics Case Review"; Agich, "Expertise in Clinical Ethics Consultation"; Baylis, "Profile of the Health Care Ethics Consultant"; Gibson, *Biases and Rationality in the Mediation Process;* Lynch, "Has Knowledge of [Interpersonal] Facilitation

Techniques"; Schwarz, *Skilled Facilitator;* Crigger, "Negotiating the Moral Order"; Gibson, "Mediation in the Medical Field."

21. Walker, M.U., "Keeping Moral Spaces Open: New Images of Ethics Consulting," *Hastings Center Report* 23 (1993):33–40, see p. 38. See also Gibson, "Mediation in the Medical Field."

22. Lipkin et al., *Medical Interview.*

23. Moreno, J.D., "Who's to Choose? Surrogate Decision-Making in New York State," *Hastings Center Report* 23 (1993):5–11.

24. ASBH report, p. 15.

25. Ibid., p. 14.

26. Fallowfield, L., Lipkin, M., and Hall, A., "Teaching Senior Oncologists Communication Skills: Results from Phase I of a Comprehensive Longitudinal Program in the United Kingdom," *Journal of Clinical Oncology* 16, no. 5 (1998):1961–68.

27. Schon, D.A. *The Reflective Practitioner: How Professionals Think in Action* (New York: Basic Books, 1983).

28. Schon, *Educating the Reflective Practitioner,* p. 6.

29. Schon, *Reflective Practitioner;* Schon, *Educating the Reflective Practitioner.*

6

Models for Ethics Consultation

Individual, Team, or Committee?

CYNDA RUSHTON, M.S.N., D.N.SC.,
STUART J. YOUNGNER, M.D., AND JOY SKEEL, B.S.N., M.DIV.

The Task Force on Standards for Bioethics Consultation endorsed an "ethics facilitation" approach for ethics consultation but was agnostic about the specific form actual consultations should take. Each of the models for delivering ethics consultation has implications for fulfilling the moral goals of the ethics facilitation approach. Yet, the reasons for employing a particular model have a great deal to do with practical issues such as the type of institution, its resources, and the specific features of the case in question. As we will see, each model has its advantages and disadvantages, and features of two different models are sometimes combined. All things being equal, however, a small team, working closely with an ethics committee, is both most practical and most likely to fulfill the goal of ethics facilitation.

Three basic models of health care ethics consultation are described in the literature: (1) individual consultant, (2) small-group consultation team, and (3) full ethics committee.[1] In this chapter we address each type, with an eye to quality in terms of accountability, continuity, and relational dimensions, as well as to how likely a particular model is to accomplish the broader goal of ethics facilitation.

Individual Consultant

The individual consultant performs the entire consultation process alone, including intake and screening, data gathering, coordination of meetings, recommendations, follow-up, documentation, and reporting. The consultant may or may not have a reporting relationship to the institutional ethics committee, and may or may not be a volunteer or paid staff member at the institution. In some instances, consultants with expertise in bioethics may be hired from an outside organization to perform ethics consultations for an institution. The training and expertise of the individual ethics consultant varies, but it is generally substantial compared with that of regular members of ethics committees or teams. Many individual consultants come from backgrounds in philosophy, theology, law, and/or medicine or nursing. Individual ethics consultants once gained their practical experience "on the job," but increasingly they are obtaining some supervised clinical experience in addition to taking traditional didactic courses and pursuing formal degrees.

The advantages of this model include its efficiency and user-friendliness. For example, the process is streamlined and is not dependent on the availability of a team of persons. It provides easier accessibility and utilization, with just a single point of contact. One person who gathers data directly may be more effective than multiple data collectors, especially since committees often receive data secondhand, and often from a potentially biased stakeholder—the involved physician. A single person who is consistently relating to the patient, family, and staff may be more likely than multiple persons to promote continuity and trust. This presumes that the individual consultant has the requisite interpersonal skills to promote communication and collaboration among the various stakeholders.

In some instances, an individual consultant may be less intimidating to those requesting ethics consultation, since discussing difficult issues is usually easier with one person than with a large group. The individual consultant may also develop relationships of trust with staff in the institution by having consistent interactions over time. This model also provides a more consistent application of knowledge and skills to the consultation process, which, in turn, may lead to greater use of ethics consultation at the institution. For these reasons, the individual consultant may be more user-friendly.

In addition, handling an increased number of consultations, as does the individual consultant, enhances his practical experience, which may improve the quality and consistency of ethics consultations. If successful, this model may result in higher visibility for the activities of the institution's ethics consultation service and may provide an avenue for the institution to make a commitment to ethics within the organization. Moreover, accountability may be enhanced in the sense that responsibility for the consultation can be traced to a single, easily identifiable individual.

Critics of the individual model argue, as does Judith Ross, that "there are values other than efficiency to be considered," and they worry about the anti-democratic potential of the individual consultant.[2] For example, when only one person gathers data about a case and leads the consultation, there is a risk that he may impose personal values or opinions on the consultation process or on other persons involved in it—a clear contravention of the ethics facilitation approach endorsed by the task force.[3] In addition, by depending on a lone individual, the process may lose the rich diversity of perspectives, disciplines, and values available in multiperson models. Even when the consultant is sensitive to these issues, blind spots about his biases and deficiencies may develop. Without involvement of others in the process, consultation may be reduced to an individual's opinion rather than an open dialogue with the goal of reaching consensus. Moreover, depending on the consultant's personality, role, and status within the institution (e.g., position as department chair), there may be a greater likelihood of coercion in the ethics consultation process.

As we said earlier, individual consultants may enhance accountability by narrowly focusing the scope of responsibility. But such accountability is largely meaningless if no one reviews the process. If the individual consultant reports to a full ethics committee, this gives a greater opportunity for scrutiny and evaluation of the process and outcome of consultation. Moreover, institutional participation, education, and "ownership" could be undermined when only one person is accountable for the entire consultation process. In this case ethics consultation could become isolated rather than incorporated into the fabric of the institution. A means for ongoing peer review along with critiques of process, knowledge, and skill will be lacking unless built into the institutional structure.

Problems will also arise if the consultant is inadequately trained or lacks the necessary skills or knowledge mentioned elsewhere in this volume. In this model there are no other resources or individuals to compensate for or enhance the collective performance of ethics consultation. If the individual consultant is not competent, respect and credibility for the consultation process may be undermined within the institution.

Despite its advantages, then, this model runs the risk of isolating the consultation process, diminishing both institutional accountability and educational opportunities. For these reasons, we think an individual consultant should have an obligation to routinely report her consultation activities to the institutional ethics committee, the administration, or governing board and to undergo performance evaluations. Regardless of her specific background and method of training, the individual consultant should have all the core competencies required for ethics consultation.[4]

Small-Group Consultation Team

In the small-group model, a team of ethics consultants, usually two to four persons, performs the consultations. Team members frequently are part of the institutional ethics committee, but teams may include others as well. Ideally, the team will include persons who represent diverse disciplines, perspectives, and values, adding a variety of skills and knowledge to the process. An institution may have more than one team so that the team "on call" can be rotated weekly or monthly. While members of an ethics consultation team will probably have different professional backgrounds and bring different knowledge and skills to the process, each member should have the basic knowledge and skills noted elsewhere.[5]

Like the individual consultant (and in contrast to a full committee), a small team has the advantages of efficiency, comfort for patients, families, and health professionals, and direct access to information. This model brings a greater diversity of perspectives and values to the consultation process than the individual model, thus placing less of a demand on any one person. When interdisciplinary teams are thoughtfully constructed, the cumulative knowledge and skills may exceed those of an individual consultant, and accountability for the ethics consultation process is likely to increase through greater institutional involvement. As team members work together, a natural peer review of the process occurs—particularly if team members communicate well with each other during the consultation and regularly debrief afterwards. An additional advantage to rotating teams is that it lessens the time required for being on call. Finally, the diversity of team members may also enhance the impartiality of the decision-making process by exposing biases and calling into question unarticulated assumptions or opinions.

Disadvantages of the small-team model include less flexibility and efficiency than the individual model (e.g., it is more difficult to assemble a team on short notice than to reach an individual). If an institution has rotating teams, the teams may vary in their competencies and their approach to ethics consultation. If a team has frequent turnover in membership, the quality of the service provided in the consultation is likely to undergo considerable fluctuation with changes in the knowledge, skill, and experience of members. Less opportunity to do consultations may lead to inexperience or a longer period to reach a level of confidence in doing consultations. As the economic realities of health care institutions increasingly demand efficient use of time, department heads and other managers may be reluctant to allow physicians, nurses, or social workers to "give" time to ethics consultation when their primary responsibility is elsewhere.

Accountability may also be a disadvantage in the small-team model, but for different reasons than the individual model. Here, accountability may be diffused by having several individuals responsible for the process. Because it is somewhat less user-friendly than the individual model, staff may become frustrated with the team approach and call for fewer consultations—even when consultations are viewed as beneficial.

Full Ethics Committee

In the full-committee model, the entire ethics committee meets together to perform consultations. One person, the committee chair, acts as facilitator. Sometimes the chair is the committee member with the most ethics "expertise." Sometimes the chair is a respected clinician with an interest in ethics. Having the full committee available for ethics consultations is likely to ensure maximal diversity in background, values, skills, and knowledge.

Most ethics committees include persons from a variety of disciplines—medicine, nursing, philosophy, theology, social work, law, and administration—and persons from the community, also with varied backgrounds. Thus, the full committee brings a diversity of personal values and backgrounds to the ethics discussion, diminishing the chance that a "philosopher king" will impose his own values. Ownership and accountability of the consultation process usually increase with the wider involvement of the institution's community that is possible with the full-committee model. Furthermore, this model has the possibility of involving the outside community by including representatives on the ethics committee. Involvement of a full committee may enhance accountability because of the clearer means to monitor and review the consultation process. Members can evaluate the process both as it is unfolding and after the consultation is completed.

The disadvantages of the full ethics committee are primarily related to its size. The large number of persons on the committee may be intimidating to patients, family members, and even staff. Even if patients or family members are invited into a committee meeting, few would argue that this is the setting for optimum communication or support. In our experience with all three models of ethics consultation, we have found that most families, house officers, and nurses are less willing and able to express their opinions in a large committee meeting. Meeting in a conference room, usually far removed from the bedside, the committee may appear as a powerful tribunal, even if that is not its mission or intent.

Members of a full committee usually do not have direct access to patients, families, staff, or medical records, and often must rely on secondhand or third-hand data presented at the committee meeting. Furthermore, problems addressed in ethics consultations usually require an ongoing process in which participants can revisit issues after new facts are gathered, new persons are involved in the process, and positions, once thought to be set in stone, have had time to evolve. Because of the size of the committee and the competing responsibilities of its members, coordination of multiple and timely meetings is difficult. Delay and absenteeism are inevitable.

With a large group, accountability may be diffused rather than focused, so "the 'buck' stops nowhere."[6] Some have cautioned about the dangers of "groupthink."[7] For example, Cassel wrote that "a committee can also provide the setting in which immoral decisions can be made for which no one has ultimate responsibility. This is most likely to occur in a setting where most persons on the committee are relatively removed from the clinical setting, where conflict of interest with administrative needs exists, and where the group dynamic is bureaucratized."[8] Finally, the advantage of the more democratic process in ethics committees may be lost, particularly if some individuals on the committee, by force of personality or position in the institutional hierarchy, dominate the discussion or impose their positions on others.

Contextual and Practical Issues

While all three models would be limited by lack of institutional resources and commitment, the individual consultant and small team probably would suffer the most, because these consultation processes are likely to be more intense, more time-consuming, and more often used. In institutions unwilling or unable (say, because of size) to support consultation activities, the full-committee model is most likely. In such cases, considerable effort should go into education of committee members. Alternatively, some institutions may choose to use their limited resources to "hire" an outside ethics consultant or to provide more education to a small group or team. Hospitals may have established traditions of individual, small team, or committee consultation that they are reluctant to change for perceived "theoretical" reasons.

Some cases lend themselves better to one model than another. For example, even when an institution employs the individual or small-team model, some cases may be best handled by full committee review. These could include:

- new or unusual cases (e.g., one for which the institution has no policy or for which an exception is being made to an existing policy);

- cases about which the individual consultant is unsure or small-team members cannot agree;
- situations that are highly controversial and have serious implications for individuals or the institution;
- cases in which patients need special protections (e.g., incompetent patients without surrogates);
- cases in which family members are challenged as legal and/or moral surrogates; and
- situations in which the ethical, legal, or social ramifications create complicated institutional risks and responsibilities.

A Mixed Model

A mixed model of ethics consultation involves some combination of the models discussed above. For example, it might involve an individual consultant or small team that reports regularly to an ethics committee, but uses the full committee in special, clearly identified circumstances. Another mixed model would be a full committee that sends out an individual committee member or a small team to gather data directly from the bedside, and then discusses the case in the full committee. An individual from the committee could return to speak with those involved in the case and to write a note in the chart. Or, an individual consultant could avail herself of respected colleagues on the full ethics committee to create an ad hoc small-team approach. Alternative models in the same institution could allow patients, families, and health professionals to choose—whether to consult an individual consultant or a full committee, for example.

Conclusion

No one model of health care ethics consultation serves every case optimally. All things being equal, we believe that a small team accountable to a larger committee is the best way to provide ethics consultation. This model maximally combines flexibility and user-friendliness with accountability and wider participation, and it is most likely to provide useful service that conforms to the ethics facilitation approach. Regardless of which model is chosen, ongoing education, evaluation, and improvement are essential. And without institutional support, *no* model will succeed.

Notes

1. See La Puma, J., and Toulmin, S.E., "Ethics Consultants and Ethics Committees," *Archives of Internal Medicine* 149 (1989):1109–12; Loewy, E.H., "Ethics Consultation and Ethics Committees," *HEC Forum* 2 (1990):351–59; Ross, J.W., "Case Consultation: The Committee or the Clinical Consultant?" *HEC Forum* 2 (1990):289–98; "HECs and Consultation" (editorial), *HEC Forum* 2 (1990):71–73; Swenson, M.D., and Miller, R.B., "Ethics Case Review in Health Care Institutions: Committees, Consultants, or Teams?" *Archives of Internal Medicine* 152 (1992):694–97; Singer, P.A., Pellegrino, E.D., and Siegler, M., "Ethics Committees and Consultants," *Journal of Clinical Ethics* 1, no. 4 (1990):263–67.

2. See Ross, "Case Consultation."

3. Society for Health and Human Values–Society for Bioethics Consultation: Task Force on Standards for Bioethics Consultation, *Core Competencies for Health Care Ethics Consultation: The Report of the American Society for Bioethics and Humanities* (Glenview, Ill.: American Society for Bioethics and Humanities, 1998), pp. 11–24

4. Ibid.

5. Ibid.

6. Singer et al., "Ethics Committees and Consultants."

7. Lo, B., "Behind Closed Doors: Promises and Pitfalls of Ethics Committees," *New England Journal of Medicine* 317, no. 1 (1987):46–50; Cassel, C., "Deciding to Forego Life-Sustaining Treatment: Implications for Policy in 1984," *Cordoza Law Review* 6 (May 1985):287–302.

8. Cassel, "Deciding to Forego Life-Sustaining Treatment."

7

The Structure and Process of Ethics Consultation Services

JOHN C. FLETCHER, PH.D., AND KATHRYN L. MOSELEY, M.D.

How should ethics consultation be structured and delivered? What norms should guide the process of consultation? We discuss these questions in the context of the ASBH report, *Core Competencies for Health Care Ethics Consultation*,[1] as well as our own experience.

We begin by discussing key elements of the structure and process of ethics consultation: access, notification, documentation, evaluation, and case review. We argue that the role of consultants as "ethics facilitators,"[2] and the goals of ethics consultation,[3] require a normative approach to these process elements. By *normative,* we mean that consultants' choices about how to conduct ethics consultations have moral implications. Furthermore, we recommend that institutions should formulate policy to safeguard the values at stake in the norms of conduct of ethics consultations. Neglect of these norms has already provoked legal action. We review some lawsuits that alleged a plaintiff's rights were violated by an ethics committee, the chair of a committee, or consultants acting for the committee. Our discussion emphasizes what ethics consultants can learn from these unfortunate cases.

Structures for Ethics Consultation

In the 1970s and early 1980s in the United States and Canada, most "ethics consultations" took place in the context of meetings of ethics committees, with the goal of resolving ethical problems or uncertainty in a particular case. In some cases—and we do not claim this was representative of all committees—the participants met in a conference room, without the patient or family members present. The chair of the committee, more often than not a physician, was a central figure in the meeting during the consultation. Some chairs acted as solo consultants for all consultations. As experience with the performance of these committees as a structure for consultation accumulated, the criticisms outweighed the praise (see Table 7.1).

TABLE 7.1. Criticisms of Ethics Consultation by Committee

- Decision making is "behind closed doors" and excludes patient or surrogate participation.[a]
- Committees are bureaucratic intrusions into the physician-patient relationship.[b]
- Committee decision making neglects key process issues and often violates patient privacy and confidentiality.[c]
- A committee approach lacks empirical evidence of benefits, especially to patients, family, or surrogates.[d]
- Ethics committees suffer from weak institutional and financial support.[e]
- Ethics committees function to replace concern for ethical issues with protection of the institution's risks of liability.[f]
- Committee members have little education and training in ethics, health care law, clinical medicine, and skills for the process of consultation.[g]
- In ethics consultation, the moral bias of a single consultant (often the chair of the committee) tends to dominate the decision-making process.[h]
- A faulty concept of "moral consensus" is at work in committee decision making.[i]

---

[a] Lo, B., "Behind Closed Doors: Promises and Pitfalls of Ethics Committees," *New England Journal of Medicine* 317 (1987):46–50.

[b] Siegler, M., "Ethics Committees: Decisions by Bureaucracy," *Hastings Center Report* 16, no. 3 (1986):263–67.

[c] Wolf, S.M., "Ethics Committees and Due Process: Nesting Rights in a Community of Caring," *Maryland Law Review* 50 (1991):798–858; Fry-Revere, S., "Some Suggestions for Holding Bioethics Committees and Consultants Accountable," *Cambridge Quarterly of Healthcare Ethics* 2 (1993):449–55.

[d] Tulsky, J.A., and Lo, B., "Ethics Consultation: Time to Focus on Patients," *American Journal of Medicine* 92 (1992):343–45.

[e] Hoffman, D.E., "Regulating Ethics Committees: Is It Time?" *Maryland Law Review* 50 (1991):746–97; Hoffman, D.E., "Evaluating Ethics Committees: A View from the Outside," *Milbank Quarterly* 71, no. 4 (1993):677–701.

[f] Annas, G.J., "Ethics Committees: From Ethical Comfort to Ethical Cover," *Hastings Center Report* 21, no. 3 (1991):18–21.

[h] Fletcher, J.C., and Hoffman, D.E, "Ethics Committees: Time to Experiment with Standards," *Annals of Internal Medicine* 120, no. 4 (1994):335–38; Fletcher, J.C., and Spencer, E.M., "Ethics Services in Health Care Organizations," in *Introduction to Clinical Ethics*, 2d ed., ed. J.C. Fletcher, P.A. Lombardo, M.F. Marshall, and F.G. Miller (Hagerstown, Md.: University Publishing Group, 1997), pp. 258–85.

[i] Scofield, G.R., "Ethics Consultation: The Least Dangerous Profession," *Cambridge Quarterly of Healthcare Ethics* 2 (1993):417–48.

[j] Moreno, J.D., "What Means This Consensus? Ethics Committees and Philosophic Tradition," *Journal of Clinical Ethics* 1, no. 1 (1990):38–43; Caws, P., "Committees and Consensus: How Many Heads Are Better than One?" *Journal of Medicine and Philosophy* 16, no. 4 (1991):375-91.

TABLE 7.2. Structures for Ethics Consultation

A. Consultation by a Team of Ethics Committee Members

   1. Interdisciplinary team of ethics committee members

   2. Ad hoc interdisciplinary team of ethics committee members and others assembled by the chair of the committee, depending on the features and dynamics of the case, to which stakeholders are to be invited

B. Ethics Consultation Service

   1. Composed of committee members and others, reporting to an ethics committee

   2. Composed of persons who are not members of an ethics committee but report to it or to another entity (e.g., the medical staff)

C. Consultation by Full Ethics Committee

D. Individual Consultants

   1. Under contract to the health care organization or ethics committee

   2. Part of a firm under contract to the health care organization

These criticisms led to experimentation with several types of structures other than closed committees in ethics consultations.[4] In this period, structural innovations had at least six aims:

1. transparency: a more open and visible process to address the criticism of "behind closed doors";
2. shared decision making: inclusion of patients and surrogates in the process and in any meetings of a committee;
3. timeliness;
4. greater protection of patients' privacy and confidentiality;
5. clinical relevance: facilitating a moral problem-solving process that has more proximity to the clinical realities than a committee deliberation; and
6. "user-friendliness": a less intimidating environment for clinicians and family members.

Today, health care organizations use one of four structures for ethics consultation (see Table 7.2). Because the degree of utilization of each type is empirically unknown, we used our impressions to rank them from A to D as most to least frequently used. Research on frequency of use is clearly needed. Our experience suggests that type A and B structures are very useful in large to mid-sized health care organizations, types C and D in small hospitals, hospice settings, and nursing homes. Other chapters in this volume discuss the strengths and weaknesses of these structures in greater detail. No one structure is proven to optimize the tasks of ethics consultation, and experimentation with structure continues. Each institution can use the type of structure most fitting for its overall size, for the way it composes teams of consultants, or for how the ethics committee might be engaged in the process of consultation.

We have observed ethics committees that use a variety of structures for ethics consultations. Where the practice is to assemble the full committee to consider cases, the committee can assign two or more consultants to prepare the case for discussion by going to the bedside, then to present the issues at a committee meeting. If the structure for the consultation is at some distance from the clinical setting, as a committee meeting must necessarily be, moving the early part of the process of moral assessment closer to the bedside improves clinical relevance and is more user-friendly for the decision makers.

The Process of Ethics Consultation

In the evolution of ethics consultation, new norms for the process emerged alongside new structures. Here we discuss the elements of the consultation process, rather than the underlying structure used to deliver this service. These process elements support the six aims discussed earlier and the social values that underlie these aims. Our discussion is a commentary on the ASBH report's section on process issues.[5]

Access to Consultation

All judgments about issues of access to health services, including consultations, draw on the ethical principle of justice as fairness. Health care organizations are morally obligated to make ethics consultations available when key decision makers have reached a moral impasse or when patient care may be seriously affected by uncertainty.

Who should have access to ethics consultations? The ASBH report supports a general standard of "open access," while recognizing that diversity among health care organizations requires different modes of adaptation to this standard. We interpret the standard to mean that any person with moral standing in a particular case ought to have access to consultation.

Ethics consultation differs from medical consultation in one major respect: frequently it is parties other than the attending physician who request the consultation. This factor can lead to friction and misunderstanding, unless the institution has a clear process for responding to requests and notifying the attending physician and patient (or surrogate) when the request has come from a different party. Physicians have legitimate concerns that ethics consultations can easily mask disagreements or other problems between attending physicians and other clinicians, including interpersonal issues. "Open access" does not mean no boundaries on who can request an ethics consultation. How should these boundaries be set? And should anyone have the authority to block an ethics consultation?

Some health care organizations restrict requests for ethics consultation to attending physicians only. We view this practice as a contradiction of a goal of ethics consultation: "to facilitate resolution of conflicts in a respectful atmosphere with attention to the interests, rights, and responsibilities of those involved."[6] Restricting access to physicians usually stems from fear and misunderstanding; worse, it conveys disrespect for the rights of patients, families, and other clinicians. Resolving an ethical problem requires the good will and effort of a small group of persons most affected by the problem, not just the physician.

The task force added to its support of a general policy of open access the opinion that "requests for consultation by patients, families, or surrogates must be honored as a matter of policy."[7] Intimidation or veiled threats (usually by physicians) against other clinicians (usually nurses) who request or wish to request an ethics consultation violate the moral ideal of open access. We discuss below a method to address the objections of an attending physician to a request for ethics consultation.

The following criterion is useful in implementing a standard of open access: any person with "moral standing" in the case may request an ethics consultation. What does this mean in practice? A test of a requester's moral standing is the degree to which that person would have a legitimate complaint if excluded from decision making. Open access clearly extends to persons with a familial relationship (including "significant others"), to anyone with a clinical relationship with the patient, and to any employee of the health care organization whose duties are morally compromised by issues in the case. A clear borderline case is when a trainee, such as a medical or nursing student, requests a consultation. We have seen instances in which such requests led to needed attention to neglected ethical issues. Nonetheless, with a policy of open access, persons who have "an axe to grind" or are manipulative can act out their motives. Consultants must carefully investigate the reasons for the request and the extent to which help from usual sources has been sought and given. Caution is advised when the requester appears to be outside the usual circle of caregivers, family, and friends. However, in our experience, requests for consultation from unusual sources (e.g., medical and nursing students, allied health professionals, administrators, custodial staff) almost always produce good results if the ethical problem in the case is of sufficient magnitude to warrant ethics consultation.

Notification and Participation

Except in emergencies, good medical and nursing practice requires notification of patients or surrogates about consultations of any type. There should be no mysterious or unwanted appearances of consultants of any type at the bedside. Breaches of this standard frequently occur in practice. Many capable patients or their surrogates leave the hospital or nursing home unaware that one or more ethics consultations affecting the patient's care have taken place. This omission is especially grievous when patients' or surrogates' participation is ethically required for decision making, but the individuals are not notified of consultations. In effect, this omission excludes them from shared decision making. The cases of *Bouvia, Bland,* and *Rideout,* discussed below, illustrate this error.

Not all consultations require notification (e.g., when two health care providers morally disagree and request help to sort out the issues and find a unified approach). Consultants must use judgment as to when to notify patients or surrogates about a request for ethics consultation and advise clinicians when this ground rule is in effect. The most obvious thresholds are when consultants must review the patient's chart and medical record to gather data and when patient's or surrogate's participation in decision making is required to seek moral consensus. Notification is not required until a request for a full consultation has been made, and consultants should not access the patient's chart without such a request and permission from the patient or surrogate.

The norm of notification raises two questions. First, who should notify whom? Ideally, the patient's physician should handle this assignment, as she should before any consultation. For the sake of timeliness, the physician can delegate this task to a clinician informed about the process of ethics consultation. Learning to carry out such assignments is a good reason for regular orientation of medical and nursing staffs to the process norms of ethics consultation. Second, what should be explained? The patient or surrogate should know that a request has been made for an ethics consultation and that trained consultants will be (1) gathering information from the patient's chart, (2) talking with the patient or surrogate and the clinicians involved in the patient's care, before (3) meeting with all parties concerned to discuss the issues.

The consultant who responds to the initial request for consultation should explain the ground rules to the person who makes the request, including the obligation to notify the patient or surrogate. If the requester is not the responsible physician, then notification of the physician should occur first to ensure her knowledge about the consultation request and involvement in decision making. In some cases, the consultant needs to notify the physician of the request for consultation as a first step in gathering information and to assist the physician with the task of notifying the patient or surrogate.

Notification safeguards the privacy of patients and surrogates. When done well, especially by the patient's physician, notification also increases the quality of the patient's or family's participation in the consultation. Appreciation that the physician has asked for help with a troubling problem can increase motivation to help. If the patient's or surrogate's participation is ethically indicated and the consultation proceeds without them, a significant violation of the family's rights will have occurred, as the *Bland* and *Rideout* cases clearly show.

Ethics consultants have no direct health care responsibility. If they review the medical record without the patient's or surrogate's knowledge, they have seriously breached the patient's privacy. Such a breach can be legally actionable, because the information in the medical record belongs to the patient.[8] In advance of any further discussion, the patient or surrogate should know that a consultation has been requested and that consultants will be reviewing the medical record to prepare for the ensuing discussions.

Failure to notify the attending physician of a request for ethics consultation seriously violates her moral and legal authority. The attending physician is morally and legally responsible for all interventions in the patient's care. This lapse occurs less frequently than failure to notify patients or surrogates, but it is no less serious. In large institutions where more than one attending physician may be caring for a patient, each attending physician should be notified.

Anyone may refuse to participate in an ethics consultation. If a patient or surrogate refuses, the consultation ought not to proceed, but the consultants may continue to support the health care team and discuss issues with them in a general manner. The practice of open access requires a reliable process to address an attending physician's refusal of ethics consultation. One approach, which avoids direct conflict between the attending physician and the consultant(s), requires the consultant to refer the attending physician to the chair of the ethics committee. The institution's policy on ethics consultation can authorize the chair to discuss with the attending physician his reasons for the refusal and to make a decision on whether the consultation should go forward. This approach assumes that only a patient or legal surrogate can veto an ethics consultation. Any clinician, especially the attending physician, can object to an ethics consultation, but he should not have the authority to block it. The institution should have a good process to address these rare objections.

Documentation and Evaluation

Ethics consultations, like all consultations, should be documented in the patient's medical record. In this matter, we differ somewhat with the task force, which recommended documentation in the medical record or "in some other permanent record."[9] The task force wished to be flexible in the face of a variety of documentation practices. "Some other permanent record" usually means that the account of the case is filed in the records of the ethics committee and may or may not be distributed to the parties to the consultation.

We prefer a "both–and" approach rather than the "either–or" approach of the task force. Good documentation requires an appropriate note in the medical record and a longer detailed account of the case suitable for evaluation and review. The goals of documentation are (1) informing all hospital staff caring for the patient of the issue(s) and important details of the consultation, (2) keeping an accurate history of all phases of the patient's care, (3) aiding in education in clinical ethics and health care law, and (4) aiding in quality assurance. To omit documentation in the medical record is to fail to seek these goals. To write only a chart note but no consultation report prevents good education and reduces quality assurance. Table 7.3 shows the elements of an adequate chart note that provides information on the end points for evaluation selected by the task force, described at the end of this section.

Hesitancy to document in the medical record usually arises from one of three causes: (1) fears of subsequent lawsuits in which the record would be discoverable, (2) failure to train consultants in writing appropriate chart notes, or (3) the marginality of consultants or the committee to clinical decision making. If such factors are evident, the remedies are to strengthen the ethics program and to educate and train consultants or the committee in better practices of documentation.

Readers should note the importance of documentation to "ethics facilitation," the preferred approach of ethics consultation as strongly endorsed by the ASBH report.[10] Consultants should not take sides or impose their moral views

TABLE 7.3. Elements of an Adequate Chart Note

- Requester and time of request
- Requester's stated concern or ethical problem(s)
- Brief synopsis of the patient's medical condition
- Who notified the patient/surrogate and attending physician
- Consultant(s) view of the ethical problem(s) in the case
- Capacity of the patient and whether advance directives exist
- Decision makers with legal and moral standing and, if such were needed, efforts to involve them
- If a meeting was required, date/time and participants
- Moral options considered and whether consensus was achieved
- If no consensus, did decision makers with legal standing resolve the question? If not, why not?
- Consultants' recommendations on the process of carrying out the consensus, if achieved.

on the decision makers in cases with two or more morally acceptable options. Good documentation of whether moral consensus was achieved and by whom is a major safeguard of this central task and a constant reminder to consultants that their role is facilitation and education.

Table 7.4 is a format for a consultation report that can be adapted to particular cases. In our view, an adequate consultation report includes the four major parts shown here: the consultant's assessment; the consultant's moral diagnosis and educational aims; goals, decision making, and implementation; and evaluation. Some numbered items in each part of the table are relevant to all cases, some would not be relevant to all. The format is worded so that parts I and II can be a consultant's "workup" for key participants to use in a meeting. Parts III and IV are worded retrospectively, a record made after such a meeting, to complete a full consultation report. The full report could be for committee review or to share with participants and the administration when the case raises policy issues.

The information gathered by following the guidelines in Tables 7.3 and 7.4 would be useful for quality assurance and for evaluation of particular consultations. For more systematic evaluation of particular consultations or an aggregate number of consultations, instruments can be designed from the end points provided by the task force.[11] Answers to the following questions would be the end points of an adequate evaluation of one or many consultations:

- Was a consensus reached?
- Who were the key decision makers?
- Was the consensus within the boundaries of social values, law, and institutional policy?
- Was the consensus implemented?
- What was the level of satisfaction among participants?

Institutional Policy on Ethics Consultation

Most health care organizations have a written policy on the mission and functions of the ethics committee. These documents typically state that ethics consultation is a committee function but are vague about standards for consultation. Organizations that offer ethics consultation can use their policy statements to identify process standards as well as other issues of competence, fairness, and accountability. Table 7.5 outlines elements for an adequate policy statement.

The policy may also recognize a place for "ethics conversations" preliminary to or alongside formal consultations. Ethical concerns of importance to clinical staff may or may not require a full consultation to explore and resolve them. We have recommended higher standards for the process of consultation. However, clinicians should not be barred from asking for information or reassurance from their ethics service. Also, ethics conversations frequently lead to full consultations and should not end without the consultant exploring the need for a consultation. Consultants can make mistakes in ethics conversations and can use these conversations as substitutes for a full consultation. Patients' privacy can also be easily breached. To guard the patient's privacy, it is best to avoid using the patient's name in the conversation or to access the patient's chart. Consultants should keep notes about their ethics conversations and report them routinely to the ethics committee.

Legal Cases Naming Ethics Committees or Consultants

To date, ethics committees or consultants have been named in five law suits and criticized by a federal judge in a sixth case. Neglect-of-process elements

TABLE 7.4. Elements of a Consultation Report

I. Consultant's Assessment

  A. What is the patient's medical condition?

    1. Identification of medical problems

    2. Diagnosis/diagnostic hypotheses

    3. Predictions and uncertainties about prognosis

      a. Prospects for full or partial recovery

      b. Is the patient terminally ill?

    4. Goals of treatment and care

    5. Any reasonable alternatives

  B. What are the relevant contextual factors?

    1. Demographic facts: age, gender, education

    2. Life situation and lifestyle of patient

    3. Family relationships

    4. Setting of care: home or institution

    5. Socioeconomic facts (e.g., insurance coverage)

    6. Language spoken

    7. Cultural factors

    8. Religion

  C. Is the patient capable of decision making?

    1. Legally incompetent (e.g., child, court determination of incompetence)

    2. Clearly incapacitated (e.g., unconscious)

    3. Diminished capacity (e.g., depression or other mental disorder interfering with understanding or judgment)

    4. Fluctuating capacity

    5. Prospects for enhancing capacity

  D. What are the patient's preferences?

    1. Understanding of condition

    2. Views on quality of life

    3. Values relevant to treatment decision making

    4. Current wishes for treatment

TABLE 7.4. *Continued*

---

    5. Advance directives

    6. Any reasons for seeking treatment regarded as medically inappropriate or refusing treatment regarded as medically indicated

  E. What are the needs of the patient as a person?

    1. Psychic suffering and possible interventions for relief

    2. Interpersonal dynamics

    3. Resources and strategies for helping the patient cope

    4. Adequacy of home environment for care of the patient

    5. Preparation for dying

  F. What are the preferences of family/surrogate decision makers?

    1. Competence as surrogate decision maker

    2. Knowledge of relevant patient preferences

    3. Opinions on quality of life of the patient

    4. Opinions on best interests of the patient

    5. Reasons for seeking treatment regarded as medically inappropriate or refusing treatment regarded as medically indicated

  G. Are there interests other than, and potentially competing with, those of the patient?

    1. Interests of family (e.g., concerns about burdens of caring for the patient, disagreements with preferences of patient)

    2. Interests of a fetus

    3. Scarce resources and competing needs for their use

    4. Interests of clinicians (e.g., professional integrity)

    5. Interests of the health care organization

  H. Are there issues of power in the interactions of the key actors in the case that need to be addressed?

    1. Between clinicians and patient/family

    2. Between patient and family

    3. Between family members/surrogates

    4. Between members of the health care team (e.g., attending physicians and house staff, physicians and nurses)

  I. Have all the parties involved in the case had an opportunity to be heard?

TABLE 7.4. *Continued*

    J. Are institutional factors contributing to moral problems posed by the case?

       1. Work routines

       2. Fears of malpractice/defensive medicine

       3. Biases favoring disproportionately aggressive treatment or neglect of treatable conditions

       4. Cost constraints/economic incentives

II. Consultant's Moral Diagnosis and Educational Aims

    A. How is the moral problem(s) in this case being framed by the participants? Does this need to be reconsidered and replaced by an alternative understanding?

    B. Identify and rank the range of relevant moral considerations.

    C. Are there relevant institutional policies pertaining to the case?

    D. Consider ethical standards and guidelines, drawing on consensus statements of commissions, interdisciplinary or specialty groups.

    E. Consider similar cases and discussions in the literature that might shed light on the analysis and resolution of moral problem(s) in the case.

    F. What are the morally acceptable options for resolving the moral problem(s) posed by the case?

III. Goals, Decision Making, and Implementation

    A. Key decision makers' considerations of the goals of treatment and care for the patient

    B. Ideas for possible interventions to meet the needs of the patient and resolve the moral problem(s)

    C. Deliberations about merits of alternative options for resolving the moral problem(s)

    D. Was a moral consensus achieved? Was it within morally acceptable boundaries?

    E. Was an acceptable plan of action negotiated and implemented?

    F. If consensus was not achieved, what did the consultant do to seek resolution? (e.g., decision makers with legal authority encouraged to resolve the issue)

IV. Evaluation

    A. Current

       1. Is the plan of action working? If not, why not?

       2. Have conditions changed in a way that suggests the need to rethink the plan?

TABLE 7.4. *Continued*

---

3. Are interactions between clinicians and the patient or surrogate helping to meet the needs of the patient, to respect the patient as a person, and to serve the goals of the plan of care?

4. Are there relevant interests, institutional factors, or normative considerations that have not been adequately addressed in planning for the care of the patient?

B. Retrospective

1. What opportunities for resolving the moral problem(s) were missed?

2. How did the care given to the patient match up to standards of good practice?

3. What factors contributed to a less than optimal resolution of the problems posed by the case?

4. Was the process of problem solving satisfactory in this case?

5. What might have been done to improve the care of the patient?

6. Are there changes in institutional policy, the clinical environment, or educational interventions that might help in preventing or better resolving moral problems posed by similar cases?

---

contributed to the causes of these suits. We briefly note the "take-home" lessons for ethics consultants from these cases, which are arranged in chronological order.

Bouvia v. Superior Court

Bouvia is the paradigmatic example of neglect of a duty to notify the patient about a consultation, as well as of the error of strongly taking sides in an ethics controversy with two morally acceptable options.[12]

In 1983, at the age of 25, Elizabeth Bouvia, a quadriplegic, refused feeding by artificial means. A lower court upheld physicians' forcefully feeding her. She became a patient at Los Angeles County High Desert Hospital in 1985. The ethics committee, apparently without dissent, supported her physicians' decision to force-feed her by a nasogastric tube. Her physicians believed that her failure to eat more was a suicidal attempt to starve herself to death. She claimed that she was eating as much as she could. A psychiatrist examined Ms. Bouvia and found her to be a capable decision maker. In 1986, a California court of appeals overturned the earlier decision and affirmed her constitutional right to refuse unwanted treatment.[13]

After the tube was removed, Ms. Bouvia and her attorney sued the hospital and the physicians for monetary damages.[14] On learning that her physicians had stated that the ethics committee was as responsible as they were, Ms. Bouvia filed an amended complaint against each member of the committee as a defendant. She did not serve the complaint against the committee members and voluntarily dropped the suit to avoid publicity.[15]

Ms. Bouvia should have been notified of the ethics committee meeting and invited to participate; she was unaware of the meeting. Consultants should always ask themselves: does the patient or surrogate know about the consultation? Have they been invited to participate? On the issues of substance in the case, the *Bouvia* court forced physicians to face the moral acceptability of the competent patient's right to refuse all unwanted treatments. The committee must have been uninformed about the consensus in the literature, described by Capron long before this conflict, on this right of competent patients.[16] The lesson for consultants is that there is no substitute for knowledge of the literature in bioethics and health care law.

In the Matter of Baby "K"

In 1992, a team from the ethics committee at Fairfax Hospital in Virginia provided consultation on the case of "Baby K." Later, a federal judge criticized the committee's faulty process and bias.[17]

At physicians' request, a team (family practice physician, psychiatrist, and minister) of the ethics committee met with Baby K's mother, who demanded life-sustaining measures for the newborn, who had anencephaly. The staff of the neonatal intensive care unit viewed these measures as futile and as violations of professional integrity. The consultants could not resolve the dispute. The team's chart note stated that care was "futile" and advised that the hospital "attempt to resolve this through our legal system" if, after a waiting period, no change occurred in the mother's position. Judge Hilton wrote in his opinion: "[Baby K's] treating physicians requested the assistance of the Hospital's 'Ethics Committee' in overriding the mother's wishes."[18]

Judge Hilton's ruling that the Emergency Medical Treatment and Active Labor Act (EMTALA) required the hospital to provide emergency ventilatory treatment for Baby K's periodic apnea (the child was by then residing in a nearby nursing home) was upheld by the Fourth Circuit Court of Appeals.[19] The U.S. Supreme Court declined to hear an appeal by the hospital, Baby K's father, and the guardian *ad litem*.

TABLE 7.5. Elements of a Policy on Ethics Consultation

---

1. Philosophy: ethically informed clinicians are the best persons to identify and resolve ethical problems with the patient and family

2. Educational program in clinical ethics and health care law to support this philosophy

3. Institutional support for education and training of ethics consultants in competencies and skills (option: cite ASBH task force report)

4. An "open policy" on who may request consultation

5. Notification of the attending physician

6. Notification of the patient or surrogate if the issue(s) ethically require his or her participation

7. A process to address physicians' objections to a consultation

8. Institutional protection for the requester

9. Guidance on documentation in the medical record

10. A statement about no charges or billing for consultation

11. Outline of accountability structure

12. Provision for evaluation of consultation and a process for complaints

---

By the time neonatologists requested consultation in this case, it may have been too late to affect the outcome. They asked the hospital ethics committee to address the mother's refusal of a DNR order, and a meeting was arranged for the next morning. However, serious lapses in process norms do raise questions about whether opportunities for a different outcome were lost in the consultation. Judge Hilton's quotation marks around "Ethics Committee" were aimed at deriding the consultants' bias in so strongly siding with physicians against the mother's position. There were also these lapses: no member of the team had discussed the issues with Baby K's mother before the meeting; Baby K's father was not notified of the meeting; and neither he nor a clergyperson of the mother's faith was included in the meeting. The mother's religious views were crucial to her insistence on treatment. She walked out of the meeting in anger over a prayer given by the minister-member of the consulting team, who envisioned Baby K's spirit "going to God."[20] In short, his prayer asserted that the baby was already dead.

The consultants' documentation in the medical record was a provocative defense of the physicians' position rather than a full moral analysis of the issues, why the effort to reach consensus failed, and the need for follow-up. No follow-up was done by the ethics team. We are also aware that, beyond their own professional training, none of the consultants had education or training for their tasks.[21] The main lesson for ethics consultants is that neglect of process issues contributed to breakdown in communication between consultants and the key decision maker. The more novel and controversial the case, the greater attention one should pay to process issues.

Bryan v. Stone et al.

In 1993, Shirley Robertson was admitted to the University of Virginia Medical Center. During the course of her treatment, the physicians involved wrote a DNR order, despite the family's objections.[22]

Bryan, the executrix of the estate of a 53-year-old patient who died at the University of Virginia (UVA) Hospital in 1993, brought two lawsuits that named the ethics committee chair and an ethics consultant (an author of this chapter, JCF), among others. The suits alleged violation of the federal EMTALA law and the Virginia Health Care Decisions Act due to use of the hospital's DNR policy, which permits physicians to write a DNR order over objections of surrogates in futility disputes. The suits were decided in UVA's favor. The federal suit resulted in an important appellate-level ruling that the EMTALA law was not relevant to this case.[23]

Early in the case, ethics consultation was refused by the family and was not a precipitating cause of the suit. The family was aggrieved because of physicians' refusals to "do everything" including vigorous resuscitation for a hopelessly ill patient. An ad hoc committee, headed by the chair of the UVA ethics committee, reviewed the case and concurred with physicians that DNR was appropriate. The report of this committee was entered into the medical record. The patient died eight days after the DNR was written. Several months later, a dispute arose between the hospital's billing department and the family. The family turned over a "final notice" to their attorneys, whose medical record review found the committee's report. The law suits ensued.

In the context of process issues, two lessons of *Bryan* stand out. First, when family members refuse an ethics consultation, an optimal effort is needed to ensure that they know how much clinicians need their participation in decision making. The family members in this case were at a considerable distance from the hospital when they refused to participate. One of us (JCF) is still unsure of how intensive the effort was to explain that their participation was needed. The second lesson is that the policy adopted by the hospital permitting a DNR order to be written over surrogates' objections in the context of futile CPR is no substitute for extraordinary efforts to mediate such disputes. Futility disputes can probably be more fruitfully resolved by community-based mediators than by any process constructed by the health care organization. Distrust of the hospital and care providers usually pervades any internal efforts at mediation.

Gilgunn v. Massachusetts General Hospital

Paris and coauthors expertly reviewed this case and its legal significance.[24]

A 72-year-old woman who was in extremely poor health and had had three previous hip replacements broke her hip in a fall. Before orthopedic surgery could occur, she had a grand mal seizure followed by many uncontrollable seizures. She had extensive brain damage and was in a coma. Her daughter, the legally authorized surrogate, informed physicians that her mother "wanted everything possible to save her life regardless of cost,"[25] and she refused to agree with the attending physician's recommendation to forgo CPR. After twenty-eight days, and still at an impasse with the surrogate, the physician requested a consultation with the hospital's Optimal Care Committee.

The Massachusetts General Hospital's ethics committee was one of the first of its type in the nation, a small group that confined its scope mainly to intensive care. The committee's chair is a psychiatrist with a longstanding practice of advocating DNR when incapacitated and hopelessly ill patients have lengthy hospital stays and family members are demanding that "everything be done."[26] The chair's note strongly advocated a DNR order to protect a hopelessly ill patient from the harms of CPR. The attending physician wrote the order and later revoked it when the daughter protested. A tracheostomy and gastrostomy tube were placed. The patient regained consciousness but was incapable of decision making.

At this stage of the case, a new attending physician assumed care. The patient then had more seizures and became unresponsive, and a number of her organ systems failed. The ICU team arranged a family meeting, which included the ethics committee and the hospital lawyer. In the midst of discussion of a DNR order, the daughter angrily walked out of the meeting. The attending physician wrote a DNR order and requested an ethics consultation. The ethics committee chairman strongly supported the rationale for writing a DNR over the daughter's objections. The attending physician repeatedly attempted to contact the surrogate, who would not speak with him. He called the family home and communicated his intent to wean the patient from the ventilator. The patient died, and her daughter sued for violations of her rights, rather than the rights of the patient. A trial court sided with the hospital.[27] The decision was on appeal, but the plaintiff withdrew shortly before the appeal went to trial.

Given the surrogate's unwillingness to discuss the issues and the chair's understanding of his role, it is unlikely that the outcome of this case could have been different. The chair's strong advocacy of only one moral option in the case challenges the basic concept of "ethics facilitation" as the preferred model of consultation advised by the task force.[28] His conduct of the consultation process approximates the example of the "authoritarian" approach discussed by the task force.[29] Alexander Capron criticized the intervention of the chair of the Optimal Care Committee, who acted not like an ethics consultant but "in the style of a medical consultant."[30] We agree with this criticism in terms of the basic understanding of process norms. Although the surrogate's position was morally controversial, it is not immoral in this society to take such a stand. Also, a hospital policy that permits a DNR to be written over a surrogate's objection should not be implemented by an ethics consultant or an ethics committee.

Ethics consultation is a practice aimed at facilitation of moral consensus. When consensus cannot be found, a process other than ethics consultation must be used to implement hospital policy. The hospital policy used in the *Bryan* case, for example, permitted the ethics committee chair to assemble an ad hoc committee of uninvolved persons to review the facts of the case and the physician's reasons for forgoing CPR in the case. Facilitation of clinicians' moral courage in writing DNR orders to prevent harm to patients is an important task for every hospital, but it is a task beyond the process of ethics consultation, which, in this case, had failed to reach consensus.

Bland, James Davis (Estate of) v. Cigna Healthplan of Texas, Inc.

The family of a patient with AIDS sued for intentional infliction of emotional harm resulting from decisions made by the chair of the hospital's ethics committee, who was also a pulmonologist, and linked to the manner of the patient's death.[31] The case was fully reported by Schwartz.[32]

The patient was a registered nurse who understood that he had a terminal illness and would die soon. In July 1993, he was admitted to Houston's Park Plaza Hospital's ICU and placed on a respirator. He was given a paralytic drug to make him comfortable, and the respirator took over his breathing function. Afraid of suffocating if he was taken off the respirator, he requested his physician to allow him to die peacefully while being ventilated. His physician agreed, and the patient soon lapsed into a coma.

The physician explained the patient's plan to the family, who understood and agreed to a DNR order on the condition that the patient remain on the respirator. Mr. Bland's physician then withdrew from the case and turned over care to a Cigna primary care physician. After a few days, the medical director of Cigna contacted the chair of the ethics committee, a pulmonologist in charge of the unit in question. The Cigna official raised questions about the patient's stay in the ICU and whether he could be moved. The chair of the ethics committee went to the unit, presumably in the role of a physician—but not the patient's physician—without consulting either the patient's original physician with whom the comfort care plan was made or the patient's family. He did discuss the care plan with the Cigna primary care physician. As a result of the intervention, the patient was removed from the respirator by a respiratory therapist and died shortly thereafter. The circumstances of Mr. Bland's death and the involvement of the pulmonologist were not discussed with the family. They learned the facts from documents prepared for another lawsuit brought by Mr. Bland's original physician against Cigna. The suit by Mr. Bland's family was settled out of court for an undisclosed amount.[33]

This case exemplifies the harmful effects of violations of norms of access, notification, and management of role conflict. In terms of access, the Cigna official did not have "moral standing" to contact the ethics committee chair for ethics consultation and should have been referred to an appropriate official. The patient's surrogate was not notified or included in the process, which likely violated Texas law.[34] The physician had a conflict of interest; he engaged in direct action while in two roles: pulmonologist and ethics committee chair. The ASBH report takes a strong position that "an individual should never serve as an ethics consultant on a case in which he/she has clinical or administrative responsibility."[35]

Rideout v. Hershey Medical Center

The *Rideout* case, involving the removal of ventilator support from a minor, also raises significant ethical questions about the role of ethics committees and consultants.

Brianne Rideout, a two-year-old patient with a brainstem glioblastoma, had undergone neurosurgery at Johns Hopkins Hospital. She was admitted to the emergency department of the Hershey Medical Center on April 6, 1992. While at Hershey, she lapsed into a stupor and required assistance to breathe. By April 13, she had a tracheostomy and was placed on a ventilator. Physicians regarded her condition as incurable, but her parents favored aggressive treatment.

Then began a period of negotiation, but no decision making about home care or hospital care. Home care was ruled out due to inadequate wiring for a ventilator. By May 20, Brianne's parents learned that her insurance coverage would soon be depleted and Medicaid was needed to cover costs. The next day, the ethics committee met at the request of the patient's physician (without the parents present) to discuss the case, and the committee supported a decision to write a DNR order. On May 22, when they were informed of this decision, the Rideouts said they were opposed, because it meant giving up on the child's life. A search began for an appropriate alternative site, without success. On July 12, the child's pupils became fixed and dilated for the first time. On July 13, her physician decided, based on discussions with the ethics committee and in the light of her deteriorating condition, to remove the ventilator.

On July 14, Brianne's physician informed the Rideouts that he would withdraw the ventilator that day. The chair of the ethics committee met with the parents to confirm the decision. Following this meeting, the parents complained to the patient advocate, who persuaded the physician and ethics committee chair to delay to allow legal consultation. Nonetheless, the removal was scheduled for 11:00 A.M. on July 15. The parents sought a judicial order to stop this action and secured the services of an attorney. The hospital had asked local police to be present to prevent disorder. While the parents were in the office of the patient advocate speaking with their attorney by phone, the physician removed the ventilator. The hospital's chaplain communicated the action to the Rideouts. Hearing this, they rushed to her room. They were described in their complaint as hysterical and crying that their daughter was being murdered. They requested that the ventilator be reconnected, but the physician declined to do so. Mr. Rideout reportedly had an acute asthma attack. The child died two days later, in the presence of her parents.

The Rideouts' eleven-count complaint raised common law, statutory, and constitutional claims, each of which the hospital contested.[36] On December 29, 1995, a three-judge panel overruled the Medical Center's challenge to claims that by stopping the ventilator over the parents' wishes, the hospital committed an assault and battery on the child, negligently and intentionally inflicted emotional distress on the parents, and impinged parental rights rooted in the free exercise of religion.[37] The panel refused to rule out punitive damages. The hospital won the arguments that it did not violate constitutional privacy and liberty interests and that EMTALA was not violated.

The panel's decision meant that the parents were free to continue their lawsuit in a jury trial. The hospital settled the case before it went to trial.

The Hershey ethics committee and its chair may have violated process norms in two respects. First, an initial meeting was held with the physician without notifying and inviting the parents. Second, the chair later met with the parents alone to inform them that the decision to withdraw ventilator support would be carried out. The chair was in this respect an agent of the physician, not the ethics facilitator that the ASBH report endorses. Two other options were available, even at that point: (1) to transfer the patient to an alternative site or, failing that, (2) to seek a court's concurrence with the decision to withdraw ventilator support. Physicians and ethics committees should not be the final arbiters of futility disputes. Nevertheless, concerns of patient suffering and dignity and the goals of medicine, coupled with the lack of timely intervention of the legal system, sometimes place physicians and ethics committees in this difficult position. Other means of mediating these disputes are critically needed until our society works out fairer approaches to allocation of expensive health care resources.

These cases illustrate the possible ill effects of neglect of good process norms in ethics consultation. Any such disputes bring ethics consultation to the attention of the legal system. One day, a court will ask directly, "For what, exactly, is an ethics consultant (or a team acting for a committee) responsible and accountable? Is there a standard of care for ethics consultation?" The correct answer to the latter is that there is no such standard in the legal sense. However, standards for an adequate process of ethics consultation are available, which health care organizations are advised to consider and voluntarily adopt to guide their practices. This chapter has discussed these standards and commends their adoption where it would be reasonable to do so.

Conclusion

We have briefly described the types of structures for ethics consultation found in health care organizations in the United States and Canada. The trend in larger institutions is away from the full ethics committee to one with fewer but more experienced consultants who can go to the bedside. Institutions may also combine elements from more than one type, such as a well-trained team of consultants composed of members of an ethics committee and others. We emphasize again that no systematic study comparing the utility of different structures has been done. However, improvement in ethics consultation can be informed by evaluating the strengths and weaknesses of how the activity is structured. Does the structure promote transparency about the purpose of ethics consultation? Does it encourage shared decision making among key stakeholders? Are consultants able to respond to requests in a timely manner? Does the structure help protect patients' privacy and confidentiality? Does it promote consultants' awareness of the most accurate information about the patient's diagnosis and prognosis?

We have devoted further discussion to standards for the process of providing ethics consultation. Those who oversee this service can ensure that the process followed in their institution fulfills certain criteria. Does the process encourage access to consultation by patients, surrogates, and others with moral standing in the case? If patients' or surrogates' participation is morally required, are they adequately notified that an ethics consultation has been requested? Are ethics consultations adequately documented in the medical record and in a form that is useful for quality improvement? Is each ethics consultation reviewed in a timely and adequate manner? Do the criteria for periodic evaluations of ethics consultations adequately reflect standards for a good process of ethics consultation?

Finally, in reporting and briefly discussing some legal disputes or judicial criticisms that named ethics committees, we have illustrated the predictable consequences of neglect of good process norms in ethics consultation. Although a standard of care in the strict legal sense is lacking, because ethics consultation is not a true profession, a court could still find one or more consultants negligent in a duty of care owed to a patient or surrogate. Based on the history of legal cases, an adverse judgment is likely to be rendered when a consultant has overstepped the boundaries of *facilitation* of ethical reflection by strongly taking sides in a dispute clearly involving more than one morally defensible option. If the plaintiff proves to a court's satisfaction that the consultant's choice led to harm or violation of the patient's rights, legal liability is clearly plausible. Such a judgment could be reinforced by a finding that neither the institution nor the consultant had considered whether to implement or adapt an appropriate response to the ASBH's recommendations on an adequate process of ethics consultation.

Acknowledgments

We acknowledge the use and adaptation of sections previously published in J.C. Fletcher, R.J. Boyle, and E.M. Spencer, "Errors in Healthcare Ethics Consultation," in *Margin of Error*, ed. S.B. Rubin and L. Zoloth (Hagerstown, Md.: University Publishing Group, 2000):343–72.

Notes

1. Society for Health and Human Values–Society for Bioethics Consultation: Task Force on Standards for Bioethics Consultation, *Core Competencies for Health Care Ethics Consultation: The Report of the American Society for Bioethics and Humanities* (Glenview, Ill.: American Society for Bioethics and Humanities, 1998).

2. Ibid., pp. 6–7.

3. Ibid., p. 8.

4. Wear, S., Katz, P., Adrzejewski, B., and Haryadi, T., "The Development of an Ethics Consultation Service," *HEC Forum* 2 (1990):75–87; Agich, G.J., and Youngner, S.J., "For Experts Only? Access to Hospital Ethics Committees," *Hastings Center Report* 21, no. 5 (1991):17–25.

5. ASBH report, pp. 9–10.

6. Fletcher, J.C., and Siegler, M., "What Are the Goals of Ethics Consultation? A Consensus Statement," *Journal of Clinical Ethics* 7, no. 2 (1996):122–26.

7. ASBH report, p. 9.

8. *Patient Health Records Privacy Act*, VA Code, sec. 32.1-127.1:03.

9. ASBH report, p. 10.

10. Ibid., pp. 6–7.

11. Ibid., p. 28.

12. The entire *Bouvia* case is well reported, except for the involvement and suit against the committee, in G.E. Pence's *Classic Cases in Medical Ethics*, 2d ed. (New York: McGraw-Hill, 1995), pp. 41–47. The court of appeals opinion is cited in L.J. Nelson's "Legal Liability of Institutional Ethics Committees to Patients," *Clinical Ethics Report* 6, no. 4 (1992):1–8.

13. *Bouvia v. Superior Court* (Glenchur), 19 Cal. App. 3d 1127, 225 Cal. Rptr. 297, 1986.

14. "Bouvia Sues Hospital Ethics Committee," *Hospital Ethics* 3, no. 1 (1987):13–14; Nelson, L.J., "Legal Liability of Institutional Ethics Committees to Patients," *Clinical Ethics Report* 6, no. 4 (1992):1–8.

15. Blades, B., and Curreri, M., "Law, Ethics, and Health Care: An Analysis of the Potential Legal Liability of Institutional Ethics Committees," *BioLaw* 2, no. 33 (1989):S317–S26; Nelson, "Legal Liability of Institutional Ethics Committees."

16. Capron, A.M., "Right to Refuse Medical Care," in *Encyclopedia of Bioethics*, ed. W.T. Reich (New York: Free Press, 1978), p. 1501.

17. *In the Matter of Baby K*, 832 F. Supp. 1022 (E.D. Va. 1993); *In "the Matter of Baby K,"* 16 F. 3d 590 (4th Cir. 1994).

18. *In the Matter of Baby K.*

19. *In "the Matter of Baby K."*

20 The Baby K. case and the ethics committee's role is discussed at length by J.C. Fletcher in "Bioethics in a Legal Forum: Confessions of an 'Expert Witness,'" *Journal of Philosophy and Medicine* 22 (1997):297–324.

21. Ibid.

22. Details of this case are based on a personal communication from the individual involved, April 20, 1994.

23. *Bryan v. Rectors and Visitors of the University of Virginia*, 95 F. 3d 349 (U.S. App. 1996).

24. Paris, J.J., Cassem, E.H., Dec, W., and Reardon, F.E., "Use of a DNR Order over Family Objections: The Case of *Gilgunn v. MGH,*" *Journal of Intensive Care Medicine* 14, no. 1 (1999):41–45.

25. Ibid.

26. Brennan, T.A., "Incompetent Patients with Limited Care in the Absence of Family Consent," *Annals of Internal Medicine* 109 (1988):819–25.

27. *Gilgunn v. Massachusetts General Hospital*, No. 92-4820 (Mass. Sup. Ct. 1995).

28. ASBH report, pp. 6–7.

29. Ibid., pp. 5–6.

30. Capron, A.M., "Abandoning a Waning Life," *Hastings Center Report* 25, no. 4 (1995):24–26.

31. *The Estate of James Davis Bland vs. Cigna Healthplan of Texas; Kenneth Lawrence Toppell, M.D.; Milton Thomas, M.D.; and Park Plaza Hospital*, In the District Court of Harris County, TX, 11th Judicial District (1995), Case No. 93-52630, No. 790732:118–19.

32. Schwartz, M., "Not What the Doctor Ordered," *Texas Monthly* (March 1995):86–89, 115–32.

33. This case is described more fully in J.C. Fletcher et al.'s *Introduction to Clinical Ethics*, 2d ed. (Frederick, Md.: University Publishing Group, 1997), pp. 271–72.

34. *Natural Death Act*, Vernon's Texas Codes Annotated 672.001 (1992); 52342 V.T.C.A. Health & Safety Code 672.001, chap. 672.

35. ASBH report, p. 30.

36. *Marlene and Tyrone Rideout v. Hershey Medical Center*, In the Court of Common Pleas, Dauphin County, PA, No. 872 S. 1995.

37. *Dauphin County Court of Common Pleas, Rideout v. Hershey Medical Center*, PICS Case No. 96-5260 (Dec. 29, 1995), J. Turgeon, Judge; Murphy, W.P., "Hospital Faces Liability for Cutting Life Support," *Pennsylvania Law Weekly* 19, no. 3 (January 15, 1996):1, 22.

8

Institutional Support for Bioethics Committees

STEVEN MILES, M.D., AND RUTH B. PURTILO, PH.D.

As outlined in preceding chapters, many aspects of ethics consultation services have institutional implications, extending far beyond their impact on the treatment of an individual patient. Indeed, these services can no more thrive without institutional support than can other essential institutional functions. But, what does it mean to support an ethics consultation service?

In this chapter we describe in practical terms the support that ethics consultation services need to meet the reasonable expectations for high-quality and accessible services; deciding to have an ethics consultation service and nominating members is not sufficient to launch a service. We highlight the relationship between the health care facility and its consultation service, focusing on three distinguishable concerns:

1. legitimizing the ethics consultation service;
2. providing infrastructure support for the service; and
3. providing administrative support to manage controversies posed by ethics consultation.

We do not address the nonclinical ethics issues (such as disclosure of capitation payment to providers) that may be brought before an ethics consultation committee.

We cannot emphasize strongly enough that the degree and nature of administrative support for each form of ethics consultation service will vary with the mission of the service, the competence of the consultants, and the size of the health care facility. For example, a committee in a small nursing home will need to know about end-of-life care, decision making for persons with compromised cognition, accommodation of personal preferences, and communication about treatment plans with local hospitals. By contrast, a committee serving a large urban hospital with obligations to indigent patients from many different cultures will benefit from learning competencies in the issues facing health care in these areas.

Legitimizing the Ethics Consultation Service

Infrastructure support for ethics committees takes material and nonmaterial forms. The health care facility must clearly legitimize the existence of the committee in the institution's clinical life. Senior administrative staff must legitimize ethics consultation by delivering a visible and unambiguous message that consultation is vital to the provision of high-quality health care and to the institution's broader mission in the community. When this authoritative support is lacking, the demise or marginalization of ethics consultation is usually inevitable, even if the finest staff members put their energies into the consultation. Senior administrators must understand the importance and role of ethics consultation and must make clear that this service is available, will function properly, and should be used appropriately by other staff.

Administrators can transmit this legitimizing message in several ways:

• Ensure that the ethics service is included in the institution's bylaws or other basic governance documents.

• Make the chair of the ethics consultation service accountable *in that role* to a senior ranking administrator. This might be the board chair, the chief executive officer, the chief operating officer, or the head of medical or nursing staff. The message to communicate is that the committee has high standing and is not a puppet or a rubber stamp for an administrative point of view on ethics problems that may arise. If the service is put under a pastoral care service in an institution with a weak pastoral care department, the committee will likely be marginalized. In complex institutions such as academic medical centers, a central ethics officer or committee with several service components in various departments may be the best solution, ensuring greater accountability and specialized expertise and access.

• Display the ethics consultation function with other central administrative functions on organizational charts, rather than buried within job descriptions. This need not mean that the ethics committee must report directly to the board or CEO, but it should have a visible presence wherever it is situated in the organization's structure. Some consultation services are located under the chief of medical staff or nursing or are divisions within existing departments. The point is to highlight that ethics consultation is a key function, akin to safety, financial management, quality assurance, or public relations.

• Recruit support for consultation from opinion shapers. An ethics service must have the support of persons who shape opinion within an institution.

Administrators should recruit that support by example, by conversation, by addressing their concerns, and by appointing respected persons to ethics consultation services or committees. All members must be able to command the respect of society, institutional peers, and patients and their families.

Infrastructure Support of the Ethics Consultation Service

Institutions must provide adequate infrastructure for the ethics committee to function. This includes the following elements: staff time; space; funds for key activities, membership training, and basic resources; and communication services, including pagers and access to libraries and web information services. The extent of infrastructure support will vary with the size of the health care facility and the mission of the consultation services.

Time

Most appointees to an ethics consultation service welcome the opportunity but sometimes become daunted by the time required for continuing service. Orientation, self-education, and meetings take time. An ethics consultation itself may take several staff hours for learning about a case, speaking with the various parties, addressing or mediating the issue, and documenting the recommendations. Evaluating the committee's work takes time, too. Members are also asked to make educational presentations to nursing, medical, administrative, and allied health staff to educate the entire staff about ethics consultation and the ethical resolution of common clinical problems.

Space

Ethics services require space: a private and uninterrupted place for confidential consultations; secure filing space for records; and an easily accessible "public" space for texts, journals, and online resources.

Financial Support

Ethics consultation is rarely a billable activity. Health care facilities must adjust productivity-based compensation so that participation in ethics consultation does not adversely affect compensation. Ethics consultation also generates personal expenses for memberships, tuition, travel, parking, and sometimes journal subscriptions, which should be reimbursed as any other administrative business expense. The institution should confirm that its liability policy specifically covers and indemnifies members of the consultation service, whether they are employees or outside consultants. Other forms of financial support may also be needed. For example, support will be required if a consultant is responsible for community education or distribution of advance directives.

Administrative Support

The institution must ensure that the ethics consultation service has an on-call schedule and that the general operator, pastors' office, and clinical areas know how to contact a consultant. The institution must also ensure access to display areas for informational materials and to teaching areas and accounts to ensure routine access to appropriate audiovisual equipment. General staff support is needed to help in the time-consuming activities of preparing schedules, gathering people together, assigning and collecting beepers, and notifying clinical staff and operators of call schedules. Such staff should be familiar with the confidential nature of the service's findings and case materials.

The administration must require each consultation service to keep records and periodically file a quality assurance report describing its progress and needs for improving health care. These reports should be grounded in the mission of the consultation service. The initial report should consist of a detailed audit of how to reconcile the consultation work with other institutional policies. For example, who, other than health professionals, may be invited to have input into the doctor-patient deliberations? Who should have access to patient's medical records and be privy to other highly sensitive patient information? Who should be allowed to make entries into the medical record? In what section of the medical record should entries be made?

Access to Information

Initially, key members of the consultation service should take one of the intensive minicourses in ethics consultation now offered by many centers. It is also valuable for at least one member to participate in a major bioethics society to get a full picture of the community of bioethics as well as current and emerging issues. Dues are usually modest and include discounts for ethics-related meetings and materials. The major societies in the United States are:

American Society for Bioethics and Humanities
4700 W. Lake Avenue
Glenview, IL 60025–1485
(847) 375–4745
www.asbh.org

The American Society of Law, Medicine and Ethics
765 Commonwealth Avenue, #1634
Boston, MA 02215–1401
(617) 262–4990
www.aslme.org

Tables 8.1 and 8.2 list major journals and information sources for ethics committees.

Administrative Management of Controversies Caused by Ethics Consultation

Institutional support must, overall, foster a climate in which those offering ethics services can carry out their work with authority and integrity in a climate free of concerns about job security, reprisals, and undue political pressure. Ethics consultation is inherently a controversial, potentially divisive, and sometimes personally threatening clinical service, and administrative support must anticipate and provide for this. A couple of features of support seem critical, as outlined below.

Whistleblower Protection

Some issues that give rise to the call for an ethics consultations may appear to challenge an institution's interests. Administrators who have legitimized the consultation service can find themselves in a defensive position with regard to the ethics consultation process. This is a stressful time for everyone. The ethics service can be permanently compromised if such a conflict of interest causes institutional pressure that inappropriately affects the advice of the consultation. The mission statement for the consultation services should explicitly state that a consultation is to put the patient's interest first.

Institutions that fail to manage a conflict between institutional interests and the clinical fiduciary duty expose themselves to serious repercussions. A widely discussed situation was the Linares case, in which a lawyer improperly advised a hospital that a father did not have authority to terminate life support for his son. The father's efforts to resolve this question were met with stonewalling and delay rather than resolution. On the eve of his son's discharge to a long-term care facility after months of hospitalization, the father held the staff back at gunpoint while he removed the life support from his son, who died. Public opinion ran strongly against the hospital.[1]

TABLE 8.1. Major ethics journals

American Journal of Law and Medicine	Published by the American Society of Law, Medicine and Ethics. Detailed reviews written by law students.
American Journal of Bioethics	A general bioethics journal published by MIT Press.
Bioethics	A general-interest academic journal for a clinical and academic audience. Published by the International Association of Bioethics.
Bioethics Forum	Practical, short, chatty, and well informed. Published by the Midwest Bioethics Center.
Cambridge Quarterly of Healthcare Ethics	A general-interest academic journal for a clinical and academic audience.
Hastings Center Report	Widely read, 30-year-old journal. Covers a variety of topics in bioethics for a broad audience.
HEC Forum	Healthcare Ethics Committee Forum. An excellent source for clinical ethics case discussion.
Journal of Clinical Ethics	A mixture of empirical studies and essays covering the core issues in bioethics.
Journal of Medical Humanities	An academic journal that focuses on the contribution of the humanities and social sciences to health care and health care education.
Journal of Medicine and Philosophy	An academic journal for bioethicists, philosophers of medicine, theologians, and religious studies scholars.
Kennedy Institute of Ethics Journal	From the Georgetown University ethics center, this general-interest academic journal aims at an informed clinical and academic audience.
Journal of Law, Medicine and Ethics	Flagship journal of the American Society of Law, Medicine and Ethics. Each issue usually explores a theme in depth.
Linacre Quarterly	Bioethics from a Catholic perspective.
Social Science and Medicine	Bioethics from the perspective of social sciences and public policy.

TABLE 8.2. Informational Services

Medline (bioethics journals) Former BioethicsLine database Kennedy Institute of Ethics Georgetown University Washington, DC 20057-1065 (202) 687-3885 www.nlm.nih.gov/databases/ databases_bioethics.html	BioethicsLine (a database now merged with Medline; see below), was a web search service covering 100 journals, newspapers, monographs, court decisions, bills, laws, and audiovisual materials; 40 indexes for citations on medicine, nursing, biology, philosophy, religion, law, and the behavioral sciences; 1973 to the present; brief abstracts of some articles. In Medline, narrow the search to "bioethics journals"; for more specific information on bioethics, use the web site listed here.
Medline National Library of Medicine 8600 Rockville Pike Bethesda, MD 20894 (800) 638-8480 www.nlm.nih.gov	The premier source for bibliographic and abstract coverage of biomedical literature. It includes 10 million records from 4,000 journals. Two-thirds of the citations have abstracts.
Kennedy Institute of Ethics Georgetown University Washington, DC 20057-1065 (800) MED-ETHX	The "human" version of the former BioethicsLine. Call the toll-free number to request a mailed response, or e-mail a request for a search using the same database as Medline. Free!
American Society for Bioethics and Humanities www.asbh.org	A professional society with links on the web.
National Institutes of Health, Bioethics Resources on the Web www.nih.gov/sigs/bioethics/	A government agency with a search engine and links.
University of Minnesota, Center for Bioethics www.bioethics.umn.edu	A university center with links.
University of Pittsburgh, Center for Bioethics and Health Law www.pitt.edu/~bioethic	A university center with links.

Policies to protect ethics service members from reprisal are essential. Administrators should disclose and discuss potential or real conflicts of interest with members of the ethics service. By this approach, leaders can foster a climate in which honest discussion of the issues is welcomed even when powerful institutional interests are at stake. In some situations, members of the ethics consultation service whose institutional roles are such that they cannot keep the patient's interest as the focus of the consultation should step aside.

Ethics consultation should be separated from personnel oversight and evaluation. For instance, we have encountered a situation in which an ethics consultant was called to assist in a clinical situation involving a patient under the care of her supervisor. There was a risk to the younger staff member in disagreeing with the position of her supervisor and a risk that the consultation could be adversely influenced by this situation. Policies must allow persons to be exempted from consultations in which they may be improperly biased or pressured. Protections against reprisal must be clear.

Focusing the Mission

Ethics consultants not only should be sheltered from personnel actions, they should not play a role in staff discipline. Ethics committees should not be responsible for oversight of impaired clinicians. They should not be providing "remedial" education to people at the request of other bodies inside or outside the institution. They should not be charged with clinical duties such as disclosing diagnoses or prognoses to patients or families.

Conclusion

Fundamentally, institutional support for ethics consultation requires a partnership between the members of the health care institution and those who have undertaken to provide this service. Strong institutional support legitimizes the consultation service and equips it to perform its work competently.

Notes

1. Miles, S., "Taking Hostages: The Linares Case," *Hastings Center Report* 19, no. 4 (1989):4.

III • QUESTIONS ON THE HORIZON

9

Organizational Ethics

Promises and Pitfalls

PAUL M. SCHYVE, M.D., LINDA L. EMANUEL, M.D., PH.D.,
WILLIAM WINSLADE, J.D., PH.D. AND
STUART J. YOUNGNER, M.D.

Clinical ethics and organizational ethics—how are they related? In attempting to answer this question, this chapter comes to the conclusion that they are perhaps inextricably intertwined. From this vantage point, we explore the implications of this relationship for the structure of ethics committees and consultation services, the application of an "ethics facilitation" approach to organizational ethics consultation, and the competencies needed by consultants in organizational ethics.

Van Rensselaer Potter, who introduced the term *bioethics* in the early 1970s, took a very broad view of its scope, as extending from the clinician-patient level (clinical ethics), through the corporate level (business and organizational ethics), to the societal and biospheric levels.[1] He saw each level as interacting with its neighbors and functioning within the context of all the other levels. Within this vision, in theory, engaging all these levels at once would be desirable—and perhaps necessary for complete success—in resolving ethical uncertainties and conflicts at any one level. But as the great baseball philosopher Yogi Berra once said, "In theory, there is no difference between theory and practice. In practice, there is."

In line with this sentiment, Robert Potter pointed out that, in practice, one must "think about bioethics globally, but act at the clinical and corporate locale to solve practical problems."[2] The Task Force on Standards for Bioethics Consultation took a similar view, focusing on the clinical level and the organizational (i.e., Van Rensselaer Potter's "corporate") level of ethical decision making, while recognizing the impact of other levels—especially the societal—on the ethical decisions that are made.

Within this narrowed context, the task force focused its attention primarily on clinical ethics, whose domain it defined as issues that arise in specific clinical cases and policies regarding patient care issues. The domain of organizational ethics was defined by the task force as an organization's positions and behavior relative to individuals (including patients, providers, and employees), groups, communities served by the organization, and other organizations. While these definitions served the task force well in focusing its findings and recommendations, our language reflects the arbitrary nature of this division. The resolution of issues that arise in specific clinical cases (clinical ethics) is often guided by an organization's positions relative to patients and providers (organizational ethics). Even an organization's expectations and support for ethical decision making at the clinical level are the result, in part, of the organization's culture: its values, its positions, and the behavior it rewards. Likewise, an organization's position on an issue (organizational ethics) may be derived from its consideration of the ethical concerns arising in the clinical domain, even in a single patient's care (clinical ethics). Within the domain of organizational ethics, the task force further recognized the lack of clear delineation between ethical decision making in "business" (sometimes called business ethics) and ethical decision making in the broader realm of an organization's "positions and behaviors."

An example may illustrate this overlap between clinical ethics and organizational ethics:

A medical director of a not-for-profit hospital is asked to approve the use of a promising but still experimental treatment for a young mother with bone cancer that has failed to respond to conventional treatments. The experimental treatment is very expensive and is not included in the patient's health plan benefits. The patient and her family have no ability to pay for the experimental treatment themselves. If it were to be provided, its cost would be absorbed by the hospital and would set a precedent for providing such treatment to other, similar patients. Just a few such exceptions would cause the hospital to delay the planned, needed upgrading of its aging cardiac ICU monitors.

It's all here: business ethics surrounding the hospital's expenditures, broader organizational ethics surrounding its policy making on the provision of experimental treatments, clinical ethics surrounding its provision of care to the individual patient. And all these ethical domains are within the context of societal ethics that balance the good of the one—this young woman—against the good of the many—the cardiac patients who will be admitted to the hospital in the future.[3]

The Separation of Clinical and Organizational Ethics

Why, when a theoretical delineation between clinical and organizational ethics breaks down in practice, as it often does, have these two domains been histori-cally separate? Why, despite the growing literature on organizational ethics,[4] does the task force—and the bioethics community in general—have more expe-rience in clinical ethics than in organizational ethics, and have more confidence in making recommendations about the core competencies for clinical ethics consultation than for organizational ethics consultation? The reasons lie in two areas, one psychological and one historical.

The first reason is that thinking about the ethical uncertainties and dilemmas holistically is not only difficult—it can be humanly impossible. In the context of a specific ethical challenge, our minds cannot consider all the potentially rele-vant factors at all the various levels—clinical, organizational, and societal—at the same time. We look for a stable context in which we can reason through our ethical uncertainty or conflict. Until recently, the organization has provided that stable context for reasoning in clinical ethics. Neither participants at the clinical level of ethical decision making nor their ethics consultants were eager to render the decision making more complex than it already was by introducing uncertainty in the organizational or societal context. In fact, participants often expected the consultant would inform those seeking consultation of the organi-zational parameters (e.g., policies) and societal parameters (e.g., law, regula-tion, and court decisions) for their decision making. Introducing "unneces-sary" uncertainty at the organizational or societal level was not a welcome role for the consultant and may have made ethical decision making at the clinical level even more of a challenge.

The second reason for this compartmentalization of clinical and organiza-tional ethics is historical. Not many years ago, three major activities in the health care system were the responsibility of three different groups of individ-uals or institutions: providing care to individuals was in the hands of clinicians; improving the health of the community—a population of people—was in the hands of public health departments and provider organizations with commu-nity missions; and managing the financing of care was in the hands of third-party payers, including the federal government, which generally reimbursed provider organizations and clinicians on a cost-plus basis.

Over the years, each of these groups developed its own strongly held ethical traditions. Clinicians made their ethical decisions within the realm of clinical ethics—with a history extending from Hippocrates, through Nuremberg, to today—that focuses on the obligation to individual patients. Public health officials and provider organizations with a community mission acted within an ethical tradition that balanced the good of the many against the good of the individual, as they spent public funds for population-focused programs such as sewers and water supplies, immunization programs, and health information campaigns and established laws for reporting and isolating communicable diseases. The boards and managers of insurance companies lived within a tradition of business ethics, including truth telling, stewardship of resources, honoring of contracts, and fiduciary responsibility to investors. These three groups conducted their separate activities within their separate ethical traditions, only infrequently generating conflicts that crossed the boundaries between these realms—the bedside, the community, and the boardroom. Thus, any conflicts among these activities, or among the three ethical traditions and their boundaries, were hidden and dormant. Only occasionally would these conflicts become the subject of an ethics consultation, and, like each of the three groups of individuals, ethics consultants could focus their attention on a single realm—that of clinical ethics.

This "division of labor" has changed quickly and dramatically. First, concerns about the rising cost of health care increased the taxpaying public's and the premium-paying employers' demands that practitioners and provider organizations be better stewards of resources, thereby mixing boardroom and bedside obligations. Second, a new form of delivery system, managed care, intentionally combined the three activities—providing care to individual patients, improving the health status of a defined (enrolled) population, and financing the care—into a single organization with a single governance and management. The theory was that by aligning these three activities, the health care system could more efficiently and cost-effectively keep a population well and treat those in its population who became sick.

Whether this theory is correct is still being debated, but in practice the combination uncovered the latent ethical conflicts between these three activities—as in the example faced by the hospital medical director described above. Unfortunately, as any health plan medical director can attest, what is considered an ethical decision within the tradition of one of these activities may be considered an unethical decision within one of the other traditions. And because these traditions have developed in separate spheres over many years, they are intensely adhered to by the three separate groups, each of which finds it hard to understand how those in the other groups can make the "unethical" decisions they do. While dialogue under these circumstances can be difficult, it cannot be avoided if ethical decisions are to be made within today's health care system. This dialogue must occur among those whose primary responsibilities lie with the bedside, community, or boardroom and by those—such as the health plan medical director—whose responsibilities span all three.

The task force concluded that no clear and absolute line can be drawn between organizational ethics, which encompasses business ethics and a community-focused mission, and clinical ethics, which focuses on the bedside. Consequently, ethics consultants will increasingly be unable to provide consultation services in one area while ignoring the other. In theory, they must address both. The question, to recall Yogi Berra's observation, is how to put the theory into practice. The task force struggled with this issue. Three areas of uncertainty arose:

1. Should today's ethics committees and consultants, whose focus has been on clinical ethics, expand to encompass organizational ethics, or should a new structure, focused on just organizational ethics, be created?
2. Is the "ethics facilitation" approach, as recommended by the task force for clinical ethics consultation, also applicable to organizational ethics consultation?
3. Regardless of the answers to these questions, what competencies should consultants in organizational ethics possess?

Each of these questions was further delineated by the task force, as discussed in the following sections.

The Structure of Ethics Committees and Consultation Services

While the task force focused its report on ethics *consultation,* it recognized that ethics committees and services, as well as individual ethicists, typically offer additional services, including education. Since clinical ethics is the ethics of care at the "bedside," it primarily affects patients and those who provide that care—doctors, nurses, and so forth. Consequently, ethics committees and services whose focus is clinical ethics tend to provide education for a subgroup of health care organization staff—the clinicians—and the strategies used for this education tend to be those most often used for health care professional education (e.g., didactic sessions, case studies). Organizational ethics, on the other hand, is more expansive in scope. It affects everyone within the organization, because it addresses interactions with payers, purchasers, visitors, the community, and other employees, as well as with patients and their families. The range of potential organizational ethical uncertainties and conflicts is almost limitless and cannot be effectively addressed through only individual case consultations or the strategies used for professional education. Rather, ethical behavior by all staff in the organization will depend on the evident values of the organization, the articulation of those values and the modeling of ethical behavior by organization leadership, and the education of staff throughout the organization.

Therefore, the education provided by ethics committees and services in organizational ethics is not limited to traditional strategies of professional education; it also includes communication strategies that maintain a high level of awareness about the importance of ethical behavior. In addition, forums for discussion of ethical uncertainty that arise in everyday work are desirable, so that the formality of consultation does not become the only mechanism for resolving the myriad uncertainties that can arise throughout the organization. And, finally, mechanisms for monitoring whether ethical guidelines are being followed throughout the organization can be put in place, to take the ethical "temperature" of the organization and to identify "hot spots" that may need leadership attention.

This difference between clinical ethics and organizational ethics suggests that if an existing clinical ethics committee or service broadens its scope to encompass organizational ethics, it will need to use new strategies for education of staff, and the employment of these new strategies—and messages—potentially requires new or expanded competencies within the committee (e.g., in marketing and communications, in human resources management, in organizational management). The ethics committee or service will also need to include within its membership individuals from the other two ethical traditions—community health and the boardroom—so that their expertise and viewpoints can become part of the committee's deliberations.

These potentially new or expanded activities, competencies, and membership should be added to an ethics committee or service that intends to address both clinical and organizational ethics. But what about consultation? Certainly the existing committee, service, or consultant has (or should have) the skills already identified in Table 1 of the ASBH report (see Appendix). These skills, which include those needed to elicit, elucidate, and facilitate resolution of value uncertainties or conflicts among various stakeholders, would be fully applicable to case consultation in organizational ethics. (The additional knowledge needed for successful organizational ethics consultation is addressed below.)

However, the task force identified two complicating factors in facilitating resolution of uncertainty or conflicts in organizational ethics. First, the party who pays for the consultation is often directly involved in the ethical conflict; in clinical ethics consultation, on the other hand, the organization's business function is usually not a party to the conflict. Second, in organizational ethics consultation, the consultant often is providing services—including ethics facilitation services—to parties that include senior leaders of the organization who have the power to influence, directly or indirectly, the consultant's status within the organization. Thus, the organizational ethics consultant may be subject to greater pressure to favor one of the parties—and potential conflict of interest— in decision making. Under these circumstances, the task force's recommendations to consultants and health care institutions become especially important:

- If the consultant has a significant relationship with a party or parties that could lead to bias, it should be disclosed.
- Individuals should not serve as a consultant for cases in which they have clinical or administrative responsibility.
- The possibility that a consultant may give advice or act against the organization's perceived financial, public relations, or other interest should be addressed proactively with the health care institution. If a specific case puts the consultant at risk with the institution, the consultant should either take the risk or withdraw from the case. If the latter, the consultant quite possibly has an obligation to suggest a replacement.
- The health care institution should create a climate in which the consultation services can be carried out with integrity (i.e., a climate free of concerns about job security, reprisals, and undue political pressure related to the ethics consultation).

This last recommendation is not easy to implement. The institution has a responsibility to provide for *effective* ethics consultation services for the institution's patients and staff—including providing for *competent* consultants. Consequently, the institution has a responsibility to evaluate the consultants' services and to improve or replace consultants who are not competent or whose efforts often lead to unsatisfactory resolution of ethical uncertainties and conflicts. The institution has an obligation, however, to determine the resolutions are "unsatisfactory" in an unbiased way, rather than only from the perspective of the institution's perceived interests. This unbiased evaluation requires the organization's leaders to support ethical decision making that respects the values of other stakeholders, not just their own. While written policies and procedures, or even contract language, can be part of this support, it ultimately depends on the leaders' understanding and commitment. The consultant can facilitate this understanding and commitment by frequently engaging the leaders in ethical discussions, so that leaders can regularly experience the role of being one of multiple stakeholders involved in reaching the decision, rather than their familiar role of ultimate decision maker.

The task force's discussions about the structure of the ethics consultation service reflected these practical considerations. Favoring creation of a unified ethics committee or service is the similarity in the skills required for facilitating resolution of ethical uncertainties and conflicts in both the clinical and organizational domains. These skills already reside (or should reside) in a clinical ethics committee or service. Also favoring a unified committee or service is the frequent overlap and interaction among clinical and organizational issues that are subject to ethical decision making—an overlap that requires a knowledge during clinical ethics consultation of organizational issues recommended in Table 2 of the ASBH report (see Appendix). Arguing against creation of a unified ethics committee or service are the special considerations (i.e., the financial and management influences) that can introduce bias into the committee's or service's actions; the expanded role of education and communication; the bewildering array of additional factors that must be considered in any decision making that spans the clinical and organizational continuum; and the perspective that is gained only through practical experience in organizational ethics and knowledge of its literature and history.

Smaller institutions (e.g., clinics, nursing homes, small hospitals) may find that separate clinical and organizational ethics structures are impractical with respect to their functioning, their costs, and their demands on participants' time. On the other hand, large organizations (such as academic medical centers), which often have compartmentalized other important functions, may conclude that separate committees or services for clinical and organizational issues are desirable because of the volume and complexity of ethical issues they face. Under this arrangement, neither the committee or service nor the organization staff should be misled into concluding that clinical and organizational ethics can be easily disentangled. Rather, the separate structures are best appreciated as the most practical way to carry out a *single* function—ethics education and consultation. That is, while the people involved and the structures may specialize, it is counterproductive to conceive of the ethics function as bifurcated. Such a misconception would not only continue to limit the dialogue, understanding, and mutual respect that must grow among those laboring at the bedside, for the community, and in the boardroom, but may also lead to unsatisfactory "resolutions" for those many ethical uncertainties and conflicts that involve both clinical and organizational issues and values. When the clinical ethics and organizational ethics structures are separate, it is critical that both formal and informal dialogue be maintained between the structures and that they work cooperatively to provide education and consultation to staff. Overlapping membership on the committees or services can facilitate this dialogue and cooperation.

Before leaving a discussion of the functional and structural relationships between clinical and organizational ethics, we need to address an additional question. What should be the functional and structural relationships between ethics committees and services and other corporate programs that relate to ethical decision making, such as corporate compliance programs (often located within the office of the general counsel), ombudsman offices, and offices of corporate integrity (often reporting to the chief executive officer or board)? Can the ethics committee or service be housed within these programs, or should they be separate? As an example of the issues to be addressed, consider corporate compliance programs.

In recent years, amid allegations of civil and criminal misconduct, many health care organizations have established corporate compliance programs to demonstrate their intent to comply with law and regulation, especially those related to financial fraud and abuse. These programs often include the setting of an ethical tone for the organization as the context for complying with law and regulation. Yet, while fraud and abuse would be considered unethical, not all violations of the law are considered ethical issues (e.g., overtime parking), nor is every action in compliance with the law considered ethical (e.g., dramatically raising prices for food and water in a disaster area). Thus, while compliance programs overlap with the scope of ethics committees and services, they do not encompass the entire scope and may include issues outside this scope. Combining a corporate compliance program with the ethics committee or service, therefore, can create confusion between ethical decision making (for which the law often provides little guidance) and compliance with the law. The former often necessitates eliciting, weighing, and reaching a balance among the differing values of multiple stakeholders; the latter is an already decided command. In addition, the heavy emphasis in a corporate compliance program on complying with regulation, and monitoring and documenting this compliance, can overshadow the broader efforts of an ethics committee or service to raise staff consciousness about the ethical implications of their decisions and actions and the process they should use (with or without a consultant's assistance) in resolving ethical uncertainty and conflict.

Nevertheless, some non–health care companies have created compliance programs in which the leaders set a strong ethical tone that discourages wrongdoing, and these leaders commit to ethical values and exemplary conduct. This tone-setting approach is distinct from a rule-oriented approach that establishes a list of dos and don'ts that fail to address the root causes of misconduct (i.e., lack of personal or corporate integrity).[5] Monitoring of compliance is integral to every compliance program, and total compliance is expected. Although clinical and organizational ethics programs include little monitoring of the implementation of ethical decisions and policies, the task force emphasized the importance of evaluating the processes and outcomes of ethics consultation for the purpose of improving the consultation services. In organizational ethics especially, policy decisions may be fully implemented in the immediate case from which they arose but, over time, may be forgotten or ignored, either because they are only infrequently invoked or because some stakeholders who were not in full agreement with the resolution subvert the policy. In addition, unlike the expectation for total compliance in corporate compliance programs, failure to follow a clinical or organizational ethics policy may be the appropriate decision, either because of unique factors in the instant case or because the context for the decision (e.g., technology, societal norms) has changed.[6] Monitoring of compliance, and capture of *variance* in compliance and the reasons for such, are necessary steps in assessing and improving the content of ethical policy and the ethical culture of the institution. Thus, a decision to unify a corporate compliance program with an ethics committee or service should be made cautiously and should consider the message conveyed to staff by the merger, the broader scope of the ethics function, and the different monitoring needs of the ethics and compliance functions. The smaller the organization, the more likely this merger can be understood by staff and can be practical and successful.

The Approach to Organizational Ethics Consultation

The task force deliberated extensively on the appropriateness of the ethics facilitation approach for organizational ethics consultation. This approach encompasses identifying and analyzing the nature of the value uncertainty that has generated the consultation and facilitating the building of consensus among the involved parties. The task force members all agreed that the ethics facilitation approach was appropriate to resolving many value-laden conflicts in organizational ethics. Certainly to the extent that a clinical ethics consultation incorporates organizational issues, the ethics facilitation approach *would* usually be used, and in many primarily organizational ethics consultations this approach *could* be used. But whether it would *always* be the best approach hinges on four factors:

1. The issues and concerns in organizational ethics are different from those in clinical ethics.
2. Identifying—and reaching—all the relevant stakeholders is more difficult than in clinical ethics.
3. Reaching consensus is likely to be more difficult than in clinical ethics.
4. Administrators have less experience in formal resolution of ethical uncertainties and conflicts than do clinicians.

The first factor—the difference in issues and concerns—reflects the relative newness of the area of organizational ethics. In the task force members' experience with clinical ethics consultation to date, few issues or concerns have arisen to which the ethics facilitation approach could not have been applied. But the full range of organizational ethics issues has not yet been subject to this empirical test, so the task force was less confident of the ethics facilitation approach's applicability to *all* organizational ethics consultations.

The second factor—identifying and reaching the stakeholders in the uncertainty or conflict—is a practical issue. The range of individuals and groups that might be affected by a decision in organizational ethics is extensive. The stakeholders in any specific ethical decision often include a patient (or more likely, patients as a group) and clinicians, just as for a decision in clinical ethics. However, in organizational ethics, parties in the other two nonbedside domains—the community and the boardroom—are also stakeholders in the decision. Thus, the organization's managers and employees, payers, employers, community members, policy makers, and even government regulators may be stakeholders.

The challenge, therefore, is to bring together the stakeholders from all three domains—even though they may be working within different ethical traditions. But in organizational ethics consultations, the participants are usually *representatives* of the interests and values of stakeholder groups, rather than the directly involved individuals (e.g., doctors, nurses, patients) in clinical ethics consultations. The more the representatives of each of the three domains and of each stakeholder group already respect each other, the more likely is the facilitation of consensus to be successful. Thus, the consultant can play a role in helping select "compatible" representatives who will exhibit mutual understanding and consensus building.

With this extended range of stakeholders, it is easy not to be aware of every potentially affected party—and some potentially affected parties may be unaware that the way in which an uncertainty or conflict is resolved may affect them. Further, recognition of the relevance of a party to the decision may come only after the decision-making process has begun—or even finished. In the ethics facilitation approach, this challenge requires the consultant to be especially vigilant to identify other parties and their needs and values, and even to represent those needs and values within the consultation process if these parties cannot join the process.[7] But when the consultant represents the needs and values of an absent party, it may be more difficult for the other involved parties to perceive the consultant as unbiased. One potential solution is to ask a third party to speak for the absent party.

The third factor—the difficulty in reaching consensus—is the consequence of the large number of stakeholders and the unmasking of value conflicts among the ethical traditions of the bedside, the community, and the boardroom (discussed above). Although these ethical traditions are not identical, there is little or no conflict among them with respect to the ethical principles they espouse. Rather, it is the relative values assigned to those principles that may conflict. For example, in the clinical relationship, the duty to the patient generally outweighs the duty to the public (a population) or to the financier of care; in the community sphere, the duty to a population generally outweighs the duty to an individual or to a financier; in the boardroom, the duty to the financier (whether investor or bondholder) is more heavily valued than the duty to an individual or to a population. Resetting the relative values to allow consensus decision making when these duties conflict is not easy, usually will not occur *within* any one tradition, and may require a societal resetting of the parameters for balancing these values. Because consensus may be unreachable in the (current) absence of society-reset parameters, ultimate decision making may need to be assigned to one individual. While it may be tempting to assign this authority to the "expert" consultant, that solution is likely to compromise the consultant's ability to facilitate discussion among the parties in the instant and future consultations; the parties will instead direct their arguments to the consultant as decision maker. In organizational ethics, the designated decision maker is often an organizational manager or administrator. When the decision to be made is especially important and contentious, the decision maker is advised to "sleep on" the intended decision a day or two in order to put the arguments in perspective (as the personalities recede) and to consult with a wise and trusted colleague before implementing it.[8]

The fourth factor—administrators' relative inexperience in the formal resolution of ethical uncertainties and conflicts—is another source of hesitation in applying the ethics facilitation approach to all organizational ethics consultations. It took time and experience for both the consultants and the seekers of consultation in clinical ethics to comfortably use an ethics facilitation approach. Organizational ethics consultants may also have to go through a developmental process, initially receiving requests for "expert" recommendations when ethical uncertainties or conflicts arise. Or, progression to an ethics facilitation approach may occur rapidly in those spheres of business in which team decision making is often employed. The relative inexperience of nonclinical administrators in engaging in formal ethical dialogue also creates anxiety among those who are currently involved in ethics consultation—the clinical ethics consultants. The consultants often believe they will initially need to provide more education and guidance to these administrators about the processes for resolving ethical uncertainties and conflict and about the traditions of clinical ethics. This anxiety may stem from both reality and bias—the latter reflecting the specifically clinical ethical tradition within which most clinical ethics consultants have trained, as well as a lingering suspicion about the "moral probity" of business.[9] The establishment of trust and mutual respect between administrators and consultants is a prerequisite to the successful use of the ethics facilitation approach in organizational ethics, especially if conducted by a unified ethics committee or service. However, when consultants assume nonfacilitative roles, such as those of "expert," "teacher," or "decision maker," the development of this trust may be inhibited.

Competencies for Organizational Ethics Consultation

Given the array of factors that must be considered in any decision making that spans the clinical and organizational continuum, the task force concluded that organizational ethics consultation will require knowledge about:

   • health care business, cost-containment, and managed care ethics, including cost shifting, billing practices, financial or administrative incentives for clinicians, resource allocation, definitions of standard or experimental care, and conflicts of interest;

- interactions with the marketplace of medicine, including the endorsement of medical products for the purposes of market promotion, and issues raised in marketing health care organizations, such as truth in advertising and promotion of unrealistic expectations;
- societal and public health obligations, including serving the medically underserved, antidumping policies, culturally sensitive care, discrimination against or by patients (e.g., based on age, race, gender, sexual orientation, religion, disability, disease, or socioeconomic status), and public disclosure of measures of organizational performance or clinical errors;
- scientific and educational health care, including institutional obligations in training future health care providers or in performing research; and
- general business issues, including relationships with employees (e.g., discrimination in hiring and promotion, conscientious objection of employees), suppliers (e.g., bidding and contracting practices), payers (e.g., cost-accounting practices), regulators (e.g., political contributions), shareholders and creditors (e.g., financial reporting), and the public (e.g., conflicts of interest in roles).

An additional area of knowledge that would be very useful in organizational ethics consultation is that of management theories and practices, including hiring and firing, reporting of misconduct, evaluation procedures, and the politics of hierarchical, horizontal, and matrixed management systems.

As is evident from this list, many of these areas of needed knowledge are distinct from those in clinical ethics, and one individual is not likely to possess both types of knowledge. Thus, in a unified or an organizational ethics committee or service, resident knowledge of all these issues may not always be a practical goal. Rather, the unified or the organizational ethics committee or service may need to satisfy these knowledge needs by other routes. First, necessary knowledge about the technical context and content of the specific ethical uncertainty or conflict under consideration is often gained in the course of the consultation itself. This requires skills in eliciting technical information from the participants and knowing how to access relevant information from other sources (e.g., experts or the literature). Second, the ethics committee or service can establish a cadre of expert consultants to whom the committee or service can turn. Third, ethics consultation (and staff education) will often require a team approach, which would encompass the necessary knowledge of both clinical and organizational ethics issues and would also model for the involved parties the respectful interplay between the knowledge bases and traditions of clinical ethics and organizational ethics. Fourth, the consultant(s) should be especially competent in, and committed to, the process of facilitating discussion and resolution of the ethical uncertainty or conflict among the relevant parties, since the consultant(s) can be less confident about having sufficient personal knowledge of the relevant technical organizational issues. Finally, both unified and organizational ethics committees or services should include a basic introduction to the knowledge areas listed above in their continuing education for committee or service members, and ethics consultants should expand their personal knowledge to include basic knowledge of these topic areas. Note that even for those who will continue to specialize in clinical ethics, basic knowledge in these organizational areas is becoming an important factor in clinical decision making.

Conclusion

As we reconsider Van Rensselaer Potter's expansive definition of bioethics,[10] we recognize that clinical ethics consultation has never really been isolated from the full circle of ethical considerations—the context of the corporate level, societal level, and biospheric level of ethical discourse. In fact, the many "clinical ethics" consultations concerning policies on patient care—encompassed by the task force's definition of clinical ethics—are really "organizational ethics" consultations, which the task force defined as encompassing an organization's position relative to individuals, including patients and providers. And, as we have argued here, in an environment of cost containment and managed care, the relevant organizational ethics now extends to the "business" aspects of health care—its financing and the stewardship of resources.

Today, therefore, resolving ethical uncertainties and conflicts in the clinical domain will require consideration and resolution of uncertainties and conflicts in other levels of the full circle of ethical considerations. These uncertainties and conflicts increasingly arise either in, or bounded by, issues at the societal level. Efforts to address these issues at the societal level are growing. The Tavistock Group is now circulating for comment "A Shared Statement of Ethical Principles for Those Who Shape and Give Health Care: A Working Draft."[11] The Institute for Ethics at the American Medical Association has embarked on a program to identify the ethical obligations of the many stakeholders in health care.[12] And, as this chapter is being written, the U.S. Congress is debating a series of measures that would, if adopted, establish a "patients' bill of rights," which would begin to set societal boundaries for resolving some of the ethical debates in health care. These activities in the public and private sectors are efforts to establish the full circle—the boundaries—in which health care decisions can be ethically made. Ethics consultants, clinicians, and administrators in health care organizations eagerly await these societal guidelines as they daily facilitate and make value-laden decisions.

Notes

1. Potter, V.R., *Bioethics: Bridge to the Future* (Englewood Cliffs, N.J.: Prentice Hall, 1971); Potter, V.R., *Global Bioethics: Building on the Leopold Legacy* (East Lansing, Mich.: Michigan State University Press, 1988).

2. Potter, R.L., "From Clinical Ethics to Organizational Ethics: The Second Stage of the Evolution of Bioethics," *Bioethics Forum* 12, no. 2 (1996):3–12.

3. Emanuel, E.J., and Emanuel, L.L., "What Is Accountability?" *Annals of Internal Medicine* 124 (1996):229–39.

4. Bishop, L.J., Cherry, N.M., and Darragh, M., *Organizational Ethics and Health Care: Expanding Bioethics to the Institutional Arena*, Scope Note 36 (Washington, D.C.: National Reference Center for Bioethics Literature, The Joseph and Rose Kennedy Institute of Ethics, Georgetown University, 1999).

5. Pell, G., "Corporate Compliance Programs: Leading Edge Practices," *Corporate Conduct Quarterly* 5, no. 3 (1997):41–43, 57.

6. Woodstock Theological Center Seminar in Business Ethics, *Ethical Issues in Managed Health Care Organizations* (Washington, D.C.: Georgetown University Press, 1999), pp. 24, 38–39.

7. Ibid., p. 22.

8. Ibid., p. 23.

9. Frederick, W.C., "The Business Ethics Question," in *Values, Nature, and Culture in the American Corporation* (New York: Oxford University Press, 1995), p. 209.

10. Potter, *Bioethics: Bridge to the Future*.

11. Tavistock Group, "A Shared Statement of Ethical Principles for Those Who Shape and Give Health Care: A Working Draft," *Effective Clinical Practice* 2 (1999):141–44.

12. Wynia, M.K., "Performance Measures for Ethics Quality," *Effective Clinical Practice* 2, no. 6 (1999):295–99; Emanuel, L.L., "Bringing Market Medicine to Professional Account," *Journal of the American Medical Association* 227 (1997):1004–5; Emanuel, L.L., "Professional Standards in Health Care," *Health Affairs* 16 (1997):52–54.

10

The Licensing and Certification of Ethics Consultants

What Part of "No!" Was so Hard to Understand?

CHARLES BOSK, PH.D.

In *Core Competencies for Health Care Ethics Consultation,* the Task Force on Standards for Bioethics Consultation (of which I was a member) had this to say about certification:

> *Voluntary Guidelines.* The Task Force unanimously recommends that the content of this report be used as voluntary guidelines. Whether these guidelines are adopted by health care organizations or education and training programs should be based on an informed discussion of the report's merits. The Task Force:
>
> • Does not wish certifying or accrediting bodies to mandate any portion of its report
>
> • Believes that certification of individuals or groups to do ethics consultation is, at best, premature
>
> • Does not intend for its report [to be] used to establish a legal national standard for competence to do ethical consultation for the reasons indicated below.[1]

"The reasons indicated below," the sparse commentary on the summary judgment, included: the possible displacement of providers and patients as "the primary decision makers at the bedside"; the potential for authoritarian approaches to ethical decision making to emerge; the implicit endorsement of the mistaken proposition that certified individuals have some special standing to engage in decision making; the undermining of disciplinary diversity within bioethics; the establishment of a substantive ethical orthodoxy that brooks no dissent; the lack of an available and reliable measure of competence; the inability of the task force to imagine such a measure; and the raft of undesired economic, political, and pragmatic consequences that would float on any administrative scheme for implementing certification. The task force, then, spends a paragraph explaining that all the problems created by certifying individuals apply to the accreditation of committees as well.[2]

The penultimate paragraph of the report explains the use of the phrase "at this time" in the sentence, "Thus, at this time, the Task Force recommends that its report be used only as voluntary guidelines."[3] The explanation is simple. "At this time" does not contemplate some later time just over the horizon when it is appropriate to make these guidelines mandatory. Rather, "at this time" is what linguists call a "hedge" term. The task force did not think that mandatory guidelines were a good idea at the time of the report's submission. The task force could not imagine that set of conditions under which mandatory guidelines would become appropriate. Yet, when the task force submitted the report, it wanted to acknowledge that, "but, of course, we may be wrong about this,"[4] so it hedged with an "at this time."

I have quoted so fully from the conclusion of the report for two reasons. First, some of the commentators on the report have discounted its plain language and insist on reading it as an opening salvo in an ongoing struggle for professional accreditation. Among these commentators are some who see the sole purpose of the task force as furthering the professionalization of bioethics. For these commentators, the fact of the task force itself was a step toward this goal. The report, with its inevitable talk of standards and guidelines, inches us along this road. From guidelines it is a short stroll to certification. At the end of the journey, bioethicists, who once celebrated their distance from the medical model and saw their work as restoring autonomy to patients and leveling the playing field for medical action, will have created a professional presence that parallels the one they once sought to displace. There are those who might even argue, task force or not, certification or not, that much of this professional co-optation of bioethics, much of this blunting of any critical thrust, has not only occurred but also had a certain inevitability about it, given the conditions under which bioethicists are routinely employed.[5] After all, as the medical historian Charles Rosenberg remarked, "Ours is a health-care system, moreover, that has consistently demonstrated the ability to incorporate the critically and morally oppositional and make it an aspect of the system."[6]

The other reason I have quoted so fully from the conclusions of the report is that I have been assigned the task of commenting on what comes after the conclusion. What does the future hold? Is certification desirable? Inevitable? Are the critics of the report right to be so skeptical of how voluntary the guidelines are intended to be? Is bioethics consultation a professional activity? If so, does that make consultants professionals? If so, what standards of accountability apply to their actions? Who enforces those standards? It is, of course, much easier to generate a cascade of questions than to formulate a few coherent answers. In this chapter, rather than lay out an answer to the question of what the future holds for bioethics consultation and bioethics consultants, I shall lay out an approach for thinking about the question. That approach focuses on two different sociological questions. Who is a professional? And how is accountability for action achieved?

Who Is a Professional?

At some level, controversy over whether the ASBH report is a step toward professionalizing ethics consultation services is most peculiar. After all, whoever provides the service, be it a physician, nurse, social worker, chaplain, psychologist, attorney, or philosopher, is a professional in some other domain. The organization in which the service is being provided is itself one that is thoroughly professionalized. So what is this debate about? How is it that ethics consultants are professionals in all their actions, save for ethics consulting? Beyond that, we need to ask, how does certifying or denying professional status to the ethics consultant affect the service being provided? What is at stake here? Why is this a label that some seek and others reject?

One way to assess this, to assess what difference it makes whether ethical consultants are considered professionals providing an expert service, is to look carefully at the social implications of work and workers being designated "professional." There are within sociology two competing perspectives on the meaning of *professional* that are germane here. Why the professionalization of ethics consulting services is so disturbing to so many becomes clear when the implications of these sociological perspectives are drawn out. In this exercise, it is important to keep in mind that although the perspectives compete within sociology, nonsociologists have no necessity to view the perspectives as alternative ways of explaining the same empirical phenomenon. Instead, the nonsociologist critic of the "professional project"[7] of bioethics can combine the perspectives in novel ways to reinforce the sense that the professionalization of ethics consultation services is an ominous development and a reversal of traditional democratic values.[8]

The sociological perspective on professionals and professional work most familiar in everyday discourse has been developed by Talcott Parsons.[9] This perspective develops a portrait of the "selfless" professional. In this view, the professional possesses expert theoretical knowledge that is acquired after a long period of adult socialization. This knowledge is then applied to solve client problems in some domain with a "high value salience" for members of the society. Here, the classic professions serve as an example of what "value salience" means concretely—medicine's domain is health; the law's, justice; and the clergy's, salvation. Without this application of expert knowledge, the client, who is described in this perspective as "incompetent," is unable to solve his or her problem.

Because, in this perspective, both professional and client share goals and values, no concern is paid to the manner in which the professional usurps the client's decision-making authority. First, since the client and professional both want the same thing—the client's return to health, the doing of justice on the client's behalf, or salvation of the client's soul—the professional is assumed to do naturally what the client wants. The assumption of value convergence makes paternalism a nonproblem. The professional's actions are simply an extension of the client's will. In this perspective, the client's seeking the professional's service is conflated with accepting the professional's plan. Second, the perspective assumes that the professional's authority to usurp client decision making is highly limited. Professional authority is not a highly generalized medium; rather, it is "functionally specific," limited to the domain of theoretical expertise. If, and when, professionals usurp lay authority, they do so only in a limited domain, as the client's agent, at the client's direction, and with the client's prior approval. A final safeguard against professionals' overreaching the legitimate sphere of their authority is their socialization in a "service ethic." It is this expectation that the professional will act as the client's fiduciary that, when combined with a faith in the superiority of expert knowledge, allows this perspective on professionals to evade the questions of individual autonomy that are so central to bioethics.[10]

Another perspective on the nature of professional authority and work grew up alongside and in opposition to the highly idealized characterization described above. Developed by Everett C. Hughes and his students,[11] this perspective develops a portrait of the "selfish" professional. In this description, all the propositions about professionals and their work that make up the model of the "selfless" professional are inverted. So instead of granting any incontestable status to expert knowledge, this perspective questions claims to expert knowledge and separates claims of theoretical knowledge from applications of that knowledge. Professions, in this view, are an organization of similarly situated workers who convince the state to provide an exclusive "license" and "mandate" to provide services. As a result of this "license" and "mandate," professionals are able to control the production of services, and through this control create an artificial scarcity and reap monopolistic benefits. The long adult period of socialization and professional codes of ethics, said by those who view professional service romantically to guarantee virtuous service to others, is viewed quite skeptically by those who emphasize the self-interested dimensions of professional behavior.

> I wish to suggest that neither sociological analysis nor public policy is well served by defining ethicality as good intentions, expressed as a formal code or as attitudes. Rather, I wish to suggest that the most useful definition does not lie in codes or in attitudes. But in behavior at work. Just as I suggested that expertise assumes empirical status according to what the expert does in his work, so I now suggest that ethicality assumes empirical status of most consequence in the ways that the ethical occupation controls the performance of work . . . *What professionals do represents their effective knowledge or expertise; how they regulate what they do in the public interest represents their effective service orientation or ethicality.*[12]

Few of the authors writing in this tradition find that the medical profession meets Freidson's test of ethicality. It is not merely that the social control of performance is lax and haphazard,[13] but also that the profession's justifications, explanations, and claims about its behavior frequently do not align with the behavior itself.

One example well illustrates the gap between the profession's claims to ethicality and its performance: namely, the ways in which information control is used to prevent patients' autonomy. This is a well-chosen example for the simplest of reasons. The empirical research reported here occurred before the institutionalization of current standards of informed consent, so this research indexes just how much of a difference bioethics has made and at the same time displays how toothless ethical codes can be in protecting patients' dignity. The earliest empirical work on the process of dying in hospitals indicated that great effort was exerted to make certain that patients did not know they were dying.[14] Physicians and, to be fair, the families of dying patients felt that such information would create untoward stress, would involve patients' "flooding out" emotionally,[15] and would, in general, make day-to-day patient management difficult.

What was true for the dying was true for other patients as well. Candor was in short supply. Physicians relied on patients' trust in the doctor's technical expertise and moral authority to guide treatment. The absence of information shared was a primary strategy of control. Fred Davis, for example, looked at how physicians manipulate uncertainty about time to recovery in order to manipulate patients. Davis sought "to distinguish between 'real' uncertainty as a clinical scientific phenomenon and the uses to which uncertainty—real or 'pretended,' 'functional' uncertainty—lends itself in the management of patients and their families by hospital physicians and other treatment personnel."[16]

Davis demonstrated that physicians and other treatment personnel feign uncertainty about the extent of and time to recovery long after such uncertainty has been resolved. This feigning of uncertainty, this dissembling, allows physicians to sustain an atmosphere of buoyant optimism, to motivate patients and their families to cooperate with arduous programs of physical therapy, and to prevent (or at least stall) patients and their families from dropping out of conventional therapy and taking up alternative therapies viewed as forms of unethical quackery by physicians who see their own evasions as ethical behavior in service of the patient's own good. Quint described the "information management practices" physicians and nurses used to avoid disclosing a breast cancer diagnosis to patients, and detailed how "both consciously and unconsciously the staff make use of strategies which limit patients' opportunity to negotiate for information."[17] Such strategies include the staff busying themselves with technical work, rotating frequently, and failing to become familiar with patients' prognoses.

In the Parsonian perspective, professional expertise subserves the physician's fiduciary relationship with the patient. In the alternative perspective, professional expertise is viewed skeptically and ironically: physicians claim to deploy their skill, expertise, and power to the patient's benefit, but a close examination of behavior shows both claims and benefits to be dubious. For our purposes here, it is not so critical to decide which perspective is more valid.[18] Rather, our concern is to point out that the actions of certified licensed practitioners can be described in terms that celebrate the profession's contribution to the collective good or that question it in quite forceful turns. In one sense, the debate over the advisability of licensure and certification is the wrong debate in which to engage. What is more important to assess is a judgment that I shall leave for others: does ethics consultation contribute to the collective good, and if so, at what cost? The questions I am prepared to discuss here are why licensure and certification is inadvisable "at this time" and why I expect "at this time" to last for a very long time indeed.

Some Practical Difficulties with Licensure and Certification

In theory, occupational licensure and certification is a consumer protection measure. Presumptively, it serves to identify for consumers practitioners whose skills and competence have met some minimal tests and standards set by the community of practitioners. In theory again, licensure and certification is particularly necessary where knowledge and skills are esoteric, where lay judgment of services is either difficult or unreliable, and where the consequences of incompetence are grave. So, while both massage therapists and vascular surgeons may receive licenses and certificates, the process of licensure and certification has a social (as well as economic) meaning for surgeons that it does not have for masseurs. Both surgeons and masseurs may properly claim to be licensed and certified professionals. Both may take pride in those claims and in the efforts required to achieve that status. But, I would argue, those claims are more consequential for the surgeon than the masseuse. One way to think about licensure and certification for an ethics consultant is to ask: does ethical consultation more closely resemble massage or surgery? Of course, when ridiculous extremes frame rhetorical questions, there is not much drama in the answer. Below, in answering as I will, I do not mean to trivialize the work of ethical consultants or that of massage therapists, or to minimize the harm that can result from a bad consultation or an incompetent massage, or to deny the benefits of either when well-executed. Rather, I wish to discuss those dimensions of everyday practice that make it likely that licensure and certification for ethics consultants holds so little promise for the protection of the public welfare, the assurance of high-quality consultation, or the prevention of consultations of dubious value.

As a collectivity of consumers, we care, and care intensely, whether vascular surgeons are licensed and certified or not. Lay standards are not sufficiently fine-grained to distinguish competent technical performance. Lay standards may establish which vascular surgeons are louts or bores and which are kind and compassionate. But a highly skilled lout in this situation may do much good, while a charming incompetent may do much harm. Unfortunately, lay standards do not provide much guidance in assessing the technical skills of the surgeon. On the other hand, while professional massage therapists undoubtedly assess performance by different criteria than do lay users of their service, it is not clear how important those technical criteria are to lay users. Clients feel that either a massage helped or it did not. Licensing and certification in this case sends a signal to lay users about what kind of service to expect; but there is little to suggest that, within the class of licensed massage therapists—that is, the class of respectable and reputable suppliers of massage—lay evaluation is inadequate.

If we knew who the clients of ethics consultants were, if we knew what the goals of consultation were, arguments for or against licensing and certification would be easier to formulate, judgments easier to make. Still, there is no reason to think that lay standards would not be adequate to judge whether the service was competently provided or not. What, then, would licensing and certification provide in the case of ethics consultants? It would for certain limit the supply of servers, creating a presumptive monopoly for those with licenses and certificates. After all, if there were licensing and certification for ethics consultants, what institution would be willing to risk the legal liabilities incurred when personnel do not meet this minimal professional standard? But while privileging the credentials of some over others, would licensing and certification do anything to promise a higher-quality service?

The difficulties with making reasonable claims for licensure and certification center on the key points of contention for assessing the nature of professional work: namely, the nature of theory, its relation to practice, and the difficulty of establishing that the occupation in question serves the public good. Let us start with theory. One can make a reasonable claim that principlism—the flexible deployment and balancing of autonomy, beneficence, nonmaleficence, and justice—is the dominant paradigm in the field.[19] However, as many have noted, knowing the principles of principlism, mastering the theory, does not necessarily provide a reliable guide to action. Two problems present themselves. First, the values of principlism are but vague guides to action. As such, they are "essentially contestable"; articulating which values should guide action is one thing, demonstrating that this or that behavior truly embodies those values is another. That one can state the principles of principlism is not necessarily a guarantee that one knows either how to recognize which situations are problematic ethically or how to choose among those principles to produce ethics in action. In addition, while principlism is the dominant paradigm in bioethics, it is by no means the only one. Competing perspectives for resolving issues include (but are not limited to) casuistry, contractarian ethics, feminist ethics, narrative ethics, a phenomenological approach, and a variety of faith-based approaches. If we as a society were to license and certify ethics consultants, would we look for mastery of principlism or would we accept mastery of other paradigms as well? Or would we look for a more general mastery, what the ASBH report identifies as "core competencies" in the skill areas of ethical assessment, group process, and interpersonal relations, and then make certain that these existed along with a core knowledge of common bioethical issues and concepts?

Whichever way we chose to assess the theoretical knowledge of the ethics consultant, we would still face a second difficulty. We would have no assurance that this theoretical knowledge, however assessed, had any relation to outcomes, good, bad, or indifferent. In part, this is so because, despite a virtual consensus that ethics consultation is a good thing, there is a lack of clarity on both how consultation should be conducted and what consultation is intended to achieve. The position that ethics consultation is desirable is one with a fair amount of institutional support at this point. Since *Quinlan*, commentators have been nearly unanimous in their dislike for using judicial arenas for resolving conflicts of medical ethics. Courts rely on procedural rules not ethical arguments, are committed to adversarial process, have no specific competence in clinical matters, are burdened with overfull dockets without taking on questions of medical ethics, and have deliberative decision-making schedules that are not geared to the needs of the instant case. The suggestion of the *Quinlan* court (the New Jersey Supreme Court) that hospitals use ethics committees to resolve cases was given some teeth when the Joint Commission on Accreditation of Healthcare Organizations specified that organizations seeking its approval need to have in place a mechanism for resolving ethical conflicts. The JCAHO is silent on what form that mechanism needs to take and on what exactly is a conflict serious enough to require its use. Nonetheless, the JCAHO's standard has spurred the development of institutional ethics committees and furthered the role of ethics consultants.[20] Similarly, the American Hospital Association has strongly urged that its member organizations have in place a process for dealing with the "inevitable" ethical conflicts that arise in everyday contexts of care.

All of this urging from courts, commentators, accrediting bodies, and professional organizations is quite clear about what institutional ethics committees and ethics consultants are to do: namely, resolve conflict. What counts as an acceptable way for accomplishing this goal, however, remains unspecified. There are numerous modes for resolving conflict that presumptively would not pass any ethical muster, for example, the simple assertion of naked power: "We will do it this way because I say so." So, while the ultimate objective of ethics consultation may be to resolve conflict, how this objective is achieved is not unimportant. How, then, are we to judge the effectiveness of ethics consultation? What measures do we use? And, if we do not have something like a community-wide consensus about how to measure the effectiveness of ethics consultation (and presumably the consultants who assume some responsibility for them) and how to think about outcomes and process, then how can we license and certify committees or consultants? In this case, we would be granting the presumptive monopoly that licensing and certification provides absent

any demonstration that any particular mode of thinking about ethical problems, any particular method of conducting consultations, yields better results
than any other. Under those conditions, it is hard to understand the grounds
for either granting or denying a license or certification to any applicant.

Some Philosophical Questions Raised by Licensure and Certification

But suppose the objections to licensing or certification stated so far either are
horribly wrong-headed (there is an agreed-upon knowledge base for clinical
ethics, a proper way to conduct an ethical consultation, and nothing mysterious
about assessing the outcome of those consultations) or have been overcome.
Let us suppose "this time" during which the task force found it inappropriate to
consider licensing and certification has come to an end and we have arrived at
some new time in which the arguments against licensing and certification have
been overcome one by one. Further, let us assume the existence of some professional body with the standing, resources, and organizational capacity to administer the requisite tests for certifying or licensing ethics consultants. To strain
the imagination just a tiny bit more, let us assume as well that we have a valid
and reliable test of the theoretical knowledge and practical skills that an ethics
consultant needs to possess.[21] Under those conditions, is licensing and certification a good idea? I obviously think not or I would not have bothered to frame
such an elaborate set of requirements that, if met, would so clearly favor licensing and certification.

After all, if there is an occupational community of ethics consultants, what
possible objection is there in its licensing and certifying its practitioners? What
possible mischief is done in informing the lay public of who meets the standards of the professional community and who does not? As I search for an
overall rationale to connect the various threats that I see in licensing and
certification, I am aware of a sputtering inchoateness in my arguments, a
quality of what about this, or that, or the next thing, that lends an air of
unwavering unreasonableness to the presentation. For this, I apologize. Yet, I
have had for some time a visceral dis-ease with the professionalization of
bioethics.[22] I can place this dis-ease in a linguistic change.

When *bioethics* denoted a substantive domain, a set of common problems
attended to by people who identified themselves as lawyers, philosophers, physicians, nurses, clergy, social workers, and social scientists and who viewed
themselves as engaged in a common interdisciplinary enterprise, I felt no great
discomfort with either the emergence of bioethics or its institutionalization in

medical centers. But now that *bioethics* denotes those very same problems, but those engaged with them, whatever their disciplinary origin, identify themselves as bioethicists, the very developments that I applauded a few years earlier now seem more ominous. The identification of *bioethicist* as a disciplinary identity seems to me to signal the closing of the social and intellectual space that the substantive concerns of bioethics had promised to open up. In short, although it may be very much too late in the game for this sort of argument to have any persuasive force, licensing and certification of ethics consultants appears to me out of step with whatever leveling, democratic impulses originally motivated bioethics. The licensing and certification of clinical ethicists appears to me an antidemocratic move that narrows who can legitimately engage the questions of bioethics, what questions can be engaged, and what answers to those questions will be accepted as valid. As others have noted, each move in the professionalization of bioethics as an applied clinical specialty has the potential to supplant lay values with expert ones, as well as the potential to shrink the zone of individual autonomy. That this potential exists in the work of those who are among the most vociferous defenders of individual autonomy in society is ironic, to say the least. Nonetheless, as Freidson suggested in the passage quoted above with regard to assessing any occupation's ethics, actions and their consequences are weightier than intentions.

So, fiery rhetoric aside, what is the specific threat to the republic that licensing and certification of ethics consultants presents to democratic order? Since this is a slippery-slope sort of argument, we have to begin with an innocent slide that should allow enough rhetorical momentum for the alleged danger to become clear. Licensing and certification implies some sort of testing; that testing involves some selection from a likely list of routine suspects—a multiple-choice fund-of-knowledge component, an essay component, a practical simulated-conundrum component, and an "assessing the character of the character" interview. Preparation for this fateful ordeal will take place through degree programs that will begin to have a more rigid structure—what we need to know and teach becomes what counts for licensure and certification.[23] Licensing and certifying exams create a "de facto" closure to the field. Those domains not featured on the exam become, in the operation of things, less important than those that are so featured. The permeable disciplinary and substantive membrane separating that which is officially bioethics from all else becomes a much finer mesh. Approaches and topics that now find a home in bioethics face the possibility of being rejected as not what we need to know, not what the licensing and certifying bodies recognize as important. To the argument that the permeability of the membrane separating bioethics from other domains is becoming more fine-grained without licensing and certification, and that this is perhaps a natural consequence of the development of intellectual maturation, academic departments, and degree-granting programs, I would have no objection. However, I would add that licensing and certification would only accelerate an undesirable process and provide less incentive to support new approaches to old questions or to explore new questions within bioethics.

Beyond all this, within a domain that has explicitly trumpeted its commitment to leveling hierarchy—especially the asymmetric decision-making authority of doctor and patient—licensing and certification creates two new elite groups: first, within the group of those licensed and certified, there are the examiners and everyone else; second, there are those with licenses and certificates and those without. Given the requirements for qualifying to even sit most licensing and certification examinations—so much course work of just this type, so many hours of just this sort of experience, so many testimonials from so many supervisors—this second elite stratifies in unintended as well as intended ways. Formal requirements are almost always legitimated rhetorically by reference to their favorable impact on standards and performance, with their resultant beneficial impact on the collective good. What advocates of formal requirements are less likely to mention is that such requirements restrict entry into a field by class, race, ethnicity, or gender. Nor are advocates forthcoming about how difficult the benefits of licensing and certification are to demonstrate.

But as baleful as are these consequences, as regrettable as is the dulling of the bioethical imagination, the loss of interdisciplinary vitality, or the formation of new elite groups, these are not the real challenge to democratic values posed by the licensing of ethics consultants. All are merely precursors, symptoms, or warning signs of the real threat posed by licensing and certification. This is a threat hard to state concisely—undoubtedly perceptive readers have by now noticed both this fact and my constant whining about it—but it is simply that the meaning of licensed and certified ethics consultants will be socially and organizationally overdetermined. That is to say, once we have licensed and certified ethics consultants, we will begin to feel that we must use them. The expert opinion will become required. As this happens, the lay voice, the values of the people, will come to be ignored. Even when the expert opinion is aligned with the lay choice, that lay choice will have no credibility or weight until ratified by the expert. And as, or if, this happens, one more domain critical to any schema of ordered liberty, one more domain that belongs in the control of ordinary, everyday people as they make life choices, ordinary and extraordinary, quotidian and unique, becomes the mystified domain of experts with specialized training, esoteric theories, fancy titles, and nicely appointed offices. When the process is complete, ordinary, everyday people lose their confidence and faith in their own ability to reason about their life choices, to know their preferences, and to make up their own minds. When the process is complete, ordinary, everyday citizens want the reassurance of an expert opinion. They become complicit in the usurpation of their own liberty. They become complicit because the presence of the licensed and certified ethics consultant has become "natural," the right thing to do. It is at this point that democratic values have become thoroughly eroded, that domination by professional expertise has become most complete. After all, those forms of social control that are most total, most pervasive, and most coercive are those that appear most "natural." It is when the need for, the legitimacy of, and the judgment by a licensed and certified ethics consultant feels most necessary that democratic values have been most eroded.[24]

In the end, licensing and certifying ethics consultants is a permanent solution to what should be seen as a temporary problem. If the need for ethics consultation is created by the need to educate doctors and patients about ways to talk with each other so that the everyday ethical problems that bedevil modern medicine can be resolved, then we can imagine a day when that education is complete, when new forms of dialogue, as well as new modes of decision making, have emerged. In this view, ethical consultants, and perhaps bioethicists, are merely transitional figures, guides as we move from old ways of conducting business in a presumably simpler time to new ways in an admittedly more complex world. But if, or when, we begin to license and certify ethics consultants, we discard this vision of bioethics as education and facilitation. We replace it with the ethics consultant as indispensable expert. This is something that, as I hope I have made clear, has the potential for much mischief.

A Temporizing Conclusion to Some Intemperate Arguments

Very early in the deliberations of the task force, we read some articles objecting to the existence and presence of ethics consultation. The arguments in these articles were forcefully stated and, in the mind of most task force members, quite extreme. During a break in our deliberations, one of the members sidled over to me and said something like, "You know if ethics consultation were done as these articles describe it, I would have the same objections. My problem is that I don't recognize ethics consulting as it is described in these articles." I imagine that many readers of this chapter have some of the same problems with my objections to licensing and certifying ethics consultants.

The ethics consulting that I have observed has been conducted by very, very decent people with the best of intentions. They work hard not to prejudge situations. They see their work as not so much making decisions as making sure that all relevant parties to a conflict have a voice and are heard. They try to make certain that all parties are aware of the full range of options. I have no doubt that, on many occasions, the mere knowledge that the disgruntled are able to seek an ethics consultation guarantees care more attentive to patients' rights than would be the case if ethics consultants were not available. I only have to think back to my fieldwork in the mid-1970s among surgeons,[25] and all those objectionable actions I observed that occurred with no public discussion, all those conflicts resolved with the simple assertion that "there are some decisions that only an attending surgeon can make," to see how much ethical consultation has changed the world for the better.

This being so, how can I object to the licensing and certification of ethical consultants, especially when the goal is merely to improve the quality of a needed service that appears to have made care more humane and promises to make it even more so in the future? Further, aware of how much good has been done by ethical consultants, how can I be so vehement—and, I must admit, that vehemence as it tumbled onto the page surprised me—and so dogmatic in my objections? In the final analysis, my objections to licensing and certification "at this time" and, to be fair, most probably at any future time, are the ones quoted at the beginning of this chapter, as stated so starkly at the conclusion of the ASBH report: the displacement of patients and providers as primary decision makers, the undermining of diversity within bioethics, the institutionalization of a particular morality, the difficulties in finding reasonable measures of competence that are then reasonably related to outcomes, and the administrative costs and consequences entailed in any schema for licensing and certification. To all those objections, I would add one more: it is hard for me to imagine that if licensing and certification were a step taken by the bioethics community that proved to be a mistaken step, we would have the capacity to recognize this mistake and correct it. Rather, I imagine us all constantly reminding ourselves that the theory and spirit of licensing and certification are quite correct, that we just need to work harder to get the practice of the thing right, that sometime soon we will get the bugs out, that we are merely at the beginning of what we all knew was going to be a difficult process. My worries, then, are less concerned with bioethics consultation, whatever its imperfections, as it is practiced now. Rather, my worries are about what ethics consultation might become under regimes of licensing and certification.

Notes

1. Society for Health and Human Values–Society for Bioethics Consultation: Task Force on Standards for Bioethics Consultation, *Core Competencies for Health Care Ethics Consultation: The Report of the American Society for Bioethics and Humanities* (Glenview, Ill.: American Society for Bioethics and Humanities, 1998), p. 31.

2. In general, there is a set of rather tendentious qualifications about the form ethics consulting takes, which I should mention here but will not. The most important of these is whether consulting is done by an individual or a committee. In general, unless stated otherwise, I assume that arguments about certification apply equally to individuals and committees. I do this fully recognizing that the licensing requirements and procedures for individuals and organizations are somewhat distinct.

3. ASBH report, p. 2.

4. Ross, J., "The Task Force Report: Comprehensible Forest or Unknown Beetles?" *Journal of Clinical Ethics* 10, no. 1 (1999):26.

5. Bosk, C.L., "Professional Ethicist Available: Logical, Secular, Friendly," *Daedalus* 128, no. 4 (1999):47–68.

6. Rosenberg, C., "Meanings, Policies, and Medicine: On the Bioethical Enterprise and History," *Daedalus* 128, no. 4 (1999):44.

7. Larsen, M.S., *The Rise of Professionalism: A Sociological Perspective* (Berkeley: University of California Press, 1979).

8. Scofield, G., "The Least Dangerous Profession?" *Cambridge Quarterly of Healthcare Ethics* 2 (1993):417–48.

9. Parsons, T., *Essays in Sociological Theory* (New York: Free Press, 1949); Parsons, T., "Professions," in *International Encyclopedia of the Social Sciences* (New York: Macmillan, 1968).

10. Crane, D., *The Sanctity of Social Life: Physicians' Treatment of Critically Ill Patients* (New York: Russell Sage Foundation, 1975).

11. Hughes, E.C., *The Sociological Eye, Book Two: Selected Papers on Work, Self, and the Study of Society* (Chicago: Aldine-Atherton, 1971); Becker, H., "The Nature of a Profession," in *Educating for the Professions* (Chicago: National Society for the Study of Education, 1962), pp. 27–46; Freidson, E., *The Profession of Medicine: A Study in the Sociology of Applied Knowledge* (1970; Chicago: University of Chicago Press, 1988); Freidson, E., *Doctoring Together* (New York: Elsevier, 1975); Goffman, E., *Asylums* (New York: Doubleday, 1961).

12. Freidson, *Profession of Medicine*, 1988 ed., pp. 360–61, emphasis in the original.

13. Freidson, E., and Rhea, B., "Processes of Control in a Company of Equals," in *Medical Men and Their Work*, ed. E. Freidson and J. Lorber (Hawthorne, N.Y.: Walter de Gruyter, 1971); Freidson, *Doctoring Together*.

14. Glaser, B., and Strauss, A., *Awareness of Dying* (Chicago: Aldine, 1965); Glaser, B., and Strauss, A., *Time for Dying* (Chicago: Aldine, 1968); Glaser, B., and Strauss, A., *Status Passages* (Chicago: Aldine-Atherton, 1971).

15. Goffman, E., *The Presentation of Self in Everyday Life* (Garden City, N.J.: Anchor-Doubleday, 1959).

16. Davis, F., "Uncertainty in Medical Diagnosis: Clinical and Functional," *American Journal of Sociology* 66 (1960):259–67.

17. Quint, J., in Freidson and Lorber, *Medical Men and Their Work*, p. 232; Quint, J., "Institutionalized Practices of Information Control," *Psychiatry: Journal for the Study of Interpersonal Processes* 28, no. 2 (1965):119–32.

18. Abbott, A., *The System of the Professions: An Essay on the Division of Expert Labor* (Chicago: University of Chicago Press, 1988). There is a third perspective on professions: namely, Abbott's "system" of professions (ibid.). This focuses on the competition among professional occupations for dominance (e.g., the struggle among psychologists, pastoral counselors, social workers, and psychiatrists for professional "jurisdiction" over mental health services). Since our concern here is less with competition between and among groups to provide a service and more with the nature of the qualifications of any individual from any occupational background, Abbott's framework is not immediately useful. However, should licensing and certification come to pass at some later date, Abbott's framework would be a useful tool for helping us understand not only why this occurred but also why whatever requirements were adopted took the shape that they did.

19. Beauchamp, T.L., and Childress, J., *Principles of Biomedical Ethics* (New York: Oxford University Press, 1979); Chambers, T., *The Fiction of Bioethics: Cases as Literary Texts* (New York: Routledge, 1999); Wolpe, P., "The Triumph of Autonomy in American Bioethics," in *Bioethics and Society: Constructing the Ethical Enterprise*, ed. R. Devries and J. Subedi (Upper Saddle River, N.J.: Prentice Hall, 1998); Hoffmaster, B., "Can Ethnography Save the Life of Medical Ethics?" *Social Science and Medicine* 35 (1992):1421–31.

20. Bosk, C.L., and Frader, J., "Institutional Ethics Committees: Theoretical Oxymoron, Empirical Black Box," in Devries and Subedi, *Bioethics and Society*.

21. The easiest objection to the hypothetical conditions I have just set for ethics consultants is that the bar has been set too high. In fact, I am making the licensing and certification of ethics consultants rest on conditions that other occupations with licensing and certification are not required to fulfill. In essence, the objection is that I have made the perfect the enemy of the good. This is indeed possible, but since I believe licensing and certification has the potential for achieving more mischief than good, I am more than willing to set very stringent criteria. I recognize that those with a sunnier view of licensing and certification are probably willing to provide less stringent criteria.

22. Bosk, C.L., *All God's Mistakes: Genetic Counseling in a Pediatric Hospital* (Chicago: University of Chicago Press, 1992), esp. chap. 6.

23. Here it is important to remember that however cynical those "grandfathered" out of the initial licensing and certification ordeal may be about how well that ordeal measures whatever we take to be core competence, the test itself will be fateful for those who have to take it: it will influence their employment opportunities, their life-chances, in real ways. If licensing and certification exams for ethical consultants take hold, and if the results of that taking hold follow the patterns of other institutionalized exam passage points in our society, we will have created three new growth industries: (1) the exam makers, graders, and administrators; (2) the exam-preparation services; and (3) the cultural critics of the whole process. As I suspect this chapter has made more than abundantly clear, I am angling for a position on the ground floor of that third line of enterprise.

24. After all this overheated prose, I think an even-minded critic might object as follows: doesn't this all depend on what the expert would recommend? That I think not is obvious. My reasons may not be so clear. Simply stated, organizing care so that ethical values and individual autonomy rely on the wisdom exercised by a professional expert embedded in a bureaucratic organization not only feels risky; it removes power and authority from the patient in order to preserve the patient's power and authority. The entire process seems to me to be filled with internal contradictions—individual autonomy is difficult to regulate bureaucratically.

25. Bosk, C.L., *Forgive and Remember: Managing Medical Failure* (Chicago: University of Chicago Press, 1979).

Core Competencies for Health Care Ethics Consultation

The Report of the American Society for Bioethics and Humanities

Editors' note: Only the text of the report is reproduced here. Copies of the full published report, including acknowledgments, table of contents, and appendixes, are available from the American Society for Bioethics and Humanities, 4700 W. Lake Avenue, Glenview, IL 60025–1485 (telephone: [847] 375–4745; email: info@asbh.org).

**Society for Health and Human Values–Society for Bioethics Consultation:
Task Force on Standards for Bioethics Consultation**

Robert M. Arnold, MD, Co-Director
University of Pittsburgh Medical Center

Stuart J. Youngner, MD, Co-Director
University Hospitals of Cleveland; Case Western Reserve University

Mark P. Aulisio, PhD, Executive Director
University of Pittsburgh

Françoise Baylis, PhD
Dalhousie University

Charles Bosk, PhD
University of Pennsylvania

Dan Brock, PhD
Brown University

Howard Brody, MD, PhD
Michigan State University

Linda Emanuel, MD, PhD
American Medical Association

Arlene Fink, PhD
University of California at Los Angeles; Arlene Fink Associates

John Fletcher, PhD
University of Virginia

Jacqueline J. Glover, PhD
West Virginia University

George Kanoti, STD
Cleveland Clinic Foundation

Steven Miles, MD
University of Minnesota

Kathryn Moseley, MD
Henry Ford Health System

William Nelson, PhD
Veterans Affairs National Center for Clinical Ethics

Ruth Purtilo, PhD
Creighton University

Cindy Rushton, DNSc, MSN
The Johns Hopkins University

Paul Schyve, MD
Joint Commission on Accreditation of Healthcare Organizations

Melanie H. Wilson Silver, MA
Society for Healthcare Consumer Advocacy of the American Hospital
Association

Joy Skeel, MDiv, BSN
Medical College of Ohio

William Winslade, PhD, JD
University of Texas Medical Branch; University of Houston

I. Introduction

What was the SHHV-SBC Task Force on Standards for Bioethics Consultation?

The Society for Health and Human Values–Society for Bioethics Consultation
(SHHV-SBC) Task Force on Standards for Bioethics Consultation included 21 scholars in the field of health care ethics, policy, and patient care. These scholars came
from a variety of professional fields including medicine, nursing, law, philosophy,
and religious studies. In addition to representatives of SHHV and SBC, representatives from the Joint Commission on Accreditation of Healthcare Organizations (JCAHO), the American Medical Association, the Society for Healthcare
Consumer Advocacy of the American Hospital Association, the Department of
Veterans Affairs, the College of Chaplains, and the American Association of Critical-
Care Nurses served on this Task Force. Funded by a grant from The Greenwall

Foundation and contributions from numerous other organizations, centers, and networks, the mission of the Task Force was to explore standards for health care ethics consultation.[1] The work of the Task Force was motivated by the belief that when patients, health care providers, or others seek the assistance of health care ethics consultants, ethics consultants should be competent to offer that assistance.

What was the focus of the Task Force?

The focus of the Task Force was health care ethics consultation. The report is divided into five main sections that: (1) define the nature and goals of ethics consultation (i.e., what ethics consultation ought to be and aim to achieve); (2) identify the types of skills, knowledge, and character traits (core competencies) that are important for conducting ethics consultations; (3) address the emerging area of organizational ethics consultation; (4) discuss the importance of evaluating ethics consultations; and (5) underscore some of the special obligations of consultants and institutions.[2]

At the outset, three points should be noted:

• Ethics committees and individual ethicists typically offer services that include education, research, policy development, and consultation. This report addresses only issues surrounding consultation.

• "Standards," for the purposes of this work, refers to the "core competencies" that the Task Force has identified as necessary for doing ethics consultation. Though there may be considerable overlap between competencies required for ethics consultation and those necessary for other ethics services, the latter are not addressed in this report.

• The report remains neutral on the question of whether ethics consultation is best performed by individuals, teams, or committees.[3]

Who is the intended audience for the report?

The report is relevant for (1) those who do ethics consultation, (2) educational programs that help to prepare individuals, teams, or committees to do ethics consultation, and (3) health care organizations that offer ethics consultation services.

How was the report developed?

The Task Force functioned as a consensus panel. It held six three-day meetings over a two-year period from May 1996 to March 1998. The major objectives of the first two meetings were to provide background information on ethics consultation and to identify issues that needed to be addressed in subsequent meetings. In meeting three and four, subcommittees met to discuss the skills, knowledge and character traits required for consultation. Competency standards and certification issues were also addressed. A preliminary report was then drafted and discussed at meeting five.

More than 1400 copies of a "discussion draft" then were distributed to various members of the bioethics community. Their feedback was collected and incorporated into a major revision of the report which was circulated and discussed by Task Force members at meeting six. A revised draft was distributed again following the meeting. A final draft was then reviewed and approved by all Task Force members. Because the Task Force was sponsored by SHHV and SBC, and included the president of the American Association of Bioethics in its membership, the report was then reviewed and adopted by the American Society for Bioethics and Humanities, the successor to these three organizations, on May 8, 1998.

For a more detailed account of the process, please see Appendix 3.

II. Core Competencies for Health Care Ethics Consultation

1. The Nature and Goals of Ethics Consultation

1.1 *Defining Ethics Consultation*

What is health care ethics consultation?

Health care ethics consultation is a service provided by an individual or group to help patients, families, surrogates, health care providers, or other involved parties address uncertainty or conflict regarding value-laden issues that emerge in health care.[4] This uncertainty or conflict may have both cognitive and affective dimensions.[5] Health care ethics consultation has two related domains, clinical ethics and organizational ethics. This report is on clinical ethics consultation, which focuses on: (1) issues that arise in specific clinical cases and (2) policy consultation regarding patient care issues (e.g., a policy concerning guidelines for life-sustaining treatment).[6] The report acknowledges the growing demand for organizational ethics consultation and discusses its relationship to clinical ethics consultation in section 3 below.

What are the typical issues that ethics consultants must be prepared to address?

Health care ethics consultants frequently help sort through the ethical dimensions of complex clinical cases. These may involve such issues as: (1) beginning of life decisions (e.g., abortion, the use of reproductive technologies), (2) end of life decisions (e.g., withholding or withdrawing treatment, euthanasia, assisted suicide), (3) organ donation and transplantation, (4) genetic testing, and (5) the spread of sexually transmitted diseases. These issues have moral and legal dimensions that may involve, among other things, patient autonomy, informed consent, competence, health care provider rights of conscience, medical futility, resource allocation, confidentiality, or surrogate decision making. The actual cases that give rise to these questions frequently also have complex interpersonal and affective features, such as guilt over a loved one's sickness or impending death, disagreement among health care providers, possible conflicts of interest, or distrust of the medical system.

Increasingly, ethical issues regarding clinical care are raised or complicated by organizational factors (see section 3 below).[7]

Due to the complexity of these ethical issues, health care providers, patients,
families, or surrogates may request assistance to help think through questions or
resolve conflicts that may be present. Typically, these ethical issues emerge in one or
more of the relationships between:

- the patient and provider (e.g., patient or provider rights, autonomy, informed
  consent, confidentiality, competence)
- the patient, the family or surrogate, and the provider (e.g., proxy decision
  making, best interest, advance directives)
- the providers (e.g., physician-nurse relationship, inter-service disputes)
  or the health care organization and the provider, patient, family and/or
  surrogate (e.g., resource allocation, do-not-resuscitate orders, discharge and
  outplacement)
- the various communities and any of the above (e.g., societal values, the intersection of a particular community's values and organizational missions, pa-
  tient/provider relationship).

In what context do these issues emerge?

These multifaceted ethical issues emerge in our society against a complex background of developing health care technologies and evolving societal, communal, institutional, professional, and individual values. Increasing racial, ethnic, and religious diversity further compounds this plurality of values. An expanding array of
possible treatments poses difficult decisions for patients, providers and the broader
community. At the same time, scarcity of resources, the need for cost containment,
and the influence of market forces raise equally complex questions about which
treatments should be available and for whom. These decisions must be made in a
pluralistic society in which individuals have the right, based on the value of autonomy, to pursue their own conception of the good. Pluralism is present in most
contemporary health care settings where a wide variety of people from different professional, cultural, and communal backgrounds are present. Since judgments concerning what "should be done" will inevitably reflect the values that underlie them,
it is easy to see how value uncertainty or even conflict can arise in this pluralistic
context. Thus, this context largely gives rise to the need for ethics consultation and,
as we discuss below, informs its role in contemporary health care settings.

*How does this context inform the role of ethics consultation in contemporary health
care settings?*

As we have seen, societal values frame the context in which ethics consultation
occurs and, therefore, shape the appropriate role for ethics consultation in contem-

porary health care settings. Individuals, for example, do not give up the right to live by their own moral values when they become patients or take up the practice of health care. These rights set boundaries that must be respected in ethics consultation, and they often suggest who has decision-making authority in different types of cases. Discussions of these boundaries, not surprisingly, comprise a large portion of the bioethics literature (e.g., explorations of informed consent, autonomy, confidentiality, privacy, resource allocation, and conscientious objection). Indeed, helping to identify the implications of these rights and who has decision-making authority in particular cases is an important role for health care ethics consultation in our society.

Societal values are often reflected in law and institutional policy, which are also part of the context that frames ethical issues that emerge in contemporary health care settings. Law and institutional policy, therefore, also inform a proper understanding of ethics consultation, and they are widely discussed in the bioethics literature. Many states, for example, have legislation that governs the application of advance directives and outlines procedures for surrogate decision making in the absence of such directives. Similarly, institutions have policies that are applicable in certain types of cases, such as guidelines on life-sustaining treatment or requests for organ or tissue donation. Helping to identify the implications of law and institutional policy for particular cases, then, is also an important role of ethics consultation in contemporary health care settings. Still, though ethics consultation must be informed by law and institutional policy, challenges to these two domains may be appropriate at times.[8]

What is the most appropriate approach to health care ethics consultation in this context?

There are a number of approaches to ethics consultation in the bioethics literature. Most of these fall between one extreme that might be termed the "authoritarian approach" and another that might be termed the "pure facilitation approach."[9] For illustrative purposes, we will briefly characterize these two extremes, point out their inadequacies, and then outline an alternate approach, "ethics facilitation," that we believe is appropriate for ethics consultation in our society. In characterizing this approach, we only describe its core features. We are not attempting to give a detailed model that will apply to every type of consultation and that excludes all other models.[10] The ethics facilitation approach is consistent with a variety of different methods and models for ethics consultation.

The authoritarian approach. The defining characteristic of the authoritarian approach to ethics consultation is its emphasis on consultants as the primary moral decision makers at the expense of the appropriate moral decision makers. Ethics consultation can be authoritarian either with respect to process or outcome. To illustrate the inadequacies of an authoritarian approach to the outcome of consultation, consider a case in which a competent well-informed adult patient refuses treatment on religious grounds (suppose the patient is a Jehovah's Witness and the treatment involves blood products). Imagine that the ethics consultant is very sensitive to the process of consultation and talks to involved parties, addressing the factual, conceptual, and normative issues raised by the case. The consultant then recommends that the patient be given treatment against his wishes, arguing that the patient's religious beliefs are false. As this case illustrates, an authoritarian approach to the outcome of consultation makes the ethics consultant the primary moral decision maker and displaces the appropriate moral decision maker, in this case the patient. This approach places the personal moral values of the ethics consultant over those of the other parties in the case. By misplacing moral decision-making authority, this approach fails to recognize the appropriate boundaries for ethics consultation, as fundamentally established by the rights of individuals in our society.

To illustrate the inadequacies of an authoritarian approach to the process of consultation, consider a case in which a family and health care team disagree over continued treatment of a critically ill adolescent. Suppose that the health care team believes that continued treatment is futile, while the family hopes for the patient's miraculous recovery. Imagine that the ethics consultant, after talking to the attending physician and reviewing the chart, sides with the health care team, and recommends that treatment be discontinued. The consultant does not reach this decision based on personal moral views, but rather from an understanding of the controversial concept of "futility" as discussed in the bioethics literature. This approach is authoritarian in its process because it excludes relevant parties from moral decision making. It fails to open lines of communication between the family and the health care team in order to work toward a consensus that falls within the boundaries set by societal values, law, and institutional policy.[11]

The pure facilitation approach. The sole goal of the pure facilitation approach is to forge consensus among involved parties. To illustrate the inadequacies of this approach, imagine that consultants facilitate a consensus between a patient's family and the health care team to override the applicable wishes of the patient as expressed in a valid advance directive. The patient has become unconscious; no other relevant new information has become known. Though the consultants are inclusive and achieve consensus, they do so without clarifying the implications of societal, legal, and institutional values for the case, which have been discussed in detail in the bioethics literature. As the case shows, by merely facilitating consensus, consultants risk forging a consensus that falls outside acceptable boundaries. In this case, the consensus amounts to a violation of the patient's right to self-determination.

The ethics facilitation approach. We believe an ethics facilitation approach is most appropriate for health care ethics consultation in contemporary society. The ethics facilitation approach is informed by the context in which ethics consultation is done and involves two core features: identifying and analyzing the nature of the value uncertainty and facilitating the building of consensus.

To identify and analyze the nature of the value uncertainty or conflict underlying the consultation, the ethics consultant must:

- gather relevant data (e.g., through discussions with involved parties, examination of medical records or other relevant documents)
- clarify relevant concepts (e.g., confidentiality, privacy, informed consent, best interest)
- clarify related normative issues (e.g., the implications of societal values, law, ethics, and institutional policy for the case)
- help to identify a range of morally acceptable options within the context.

Health care ethics consultants also should help to address the value uncertainty or conflict by facilitating the building of consensus among involved parties (e.g., patients, families, surrogates, health care providers).[12] This requires them to:

- ensure that involved parties have their voices heard
- assist involved individuals in clarifying their own values
- help facilitate the building of morally acceptable shared commitments or understandings within the context.

In contrast to the other approaches, the ethics facilitation approach recognizes the boundaries for morally acceptable solutions normally set by the context in which ethics consultation is done. In contrast to the authoritarian approach, ethics facilitation emphasizes an inclusive consensus-building process. It respects the rights of individuals to live by their own moral values by not misplacing moral decision-making authority or acceding to the personal moral views of the consultant. In contrast to the pure facilitation approach, ethics facilitation recognizes that societal values, law, and institutional policy, often as discussed in the bioethics literature, have implications for a morally acceptable consensus. The ethics facilitation approach is fundamentally consistent with the rights of individuals to live by their own moral values and the fact of pluralism. It, therefore, responds to the need for ethics consultation as it emerges in our society.

What is the role for ethics consultants in guiding discussion among morally acceptable options?

Some cases will have a number of options that are acceptable to involved parties. This raises the question of what role consultants may play in guiding discussion among these options, especially when they see a particular option as optimal. Suppose, for example, that a competent terminally ill patient clearly expresses the wish to have life-sustaining treatment withdrawn. The patient's family is not willing to "give up" and pressures the patient to continue the treatment. The patient will wait for a time before having treatment withdrawn in order to appease the family, but really does not want to do so.

It would appear, then, that there are at least two morally acceptable options in the case. The consultant may wish to discuss with the family the importance of having the patient's values respected. The consultant may guide discussion here in a way that enhances the decision-making authority of the patient which is well established by societal values and law (and presumably by institutional policy as well) and confirmed in the bioethics literature.

Suppose, however, that in the above case, the ethics consultant shares the personal moral values of the patient: Treatment should be withdrawn because longer life is not desirable under the circumstances. It is impossible for ethics consultants to be value neutral. Consultants will typically have their own moral views about the issues in case consultations and about how cases would be best resolved. These views will inevitably influence their consultation work. We think that it is important that consultants make it clear to other involved parties both when they are offering moral judgments based on their own values and the reasons underlying their position. The line between guiding and driving discussion is very difficult to draw, much like the line between persuasion and manipulation in informed-consent discussions. Ethics consultants, then, need to be sensitive to this and should not usurp moral decision-making authority or impose their values on other involved parties. This requires that consultants be able to identify and articulate their own moral views and develop self-awareness regarding how their views affect consultation.

What if consensus among the involved parties cannot be reached?

When asked to provide guidance in what seems like an intractable conflict, consultants, by using facilitation, mediation or other conflict resolution techniques, can often help involved parties come to a mutually agreeable solution. For example, conflict can sometimes be resolved by ensuring that all participants have a similar understanding of the clinical facts, bringing in outside persons who might be able to elucidate cultural or religious values, or brainstorming to develop alternative solutions.

Unfortunately, in some cases a consensus cannot be reached. Where consensus cannot be reached, the proper course of action can sometimes be determined by answering the question "Who should be allowed to make the decision?" Societal values often indicate who should be allowed to make the decision in the absence of consensus. As several of the cases above underscore, the right of a competent and well-informed patient to refuse treatment typically establishes decision-making authority even if some family members or health care providers disagree with the decision. Similarly, the right of conscientious objection typically gives a health care provider the authority to refuse to participate in a procedure that would seriously violate his or her conscience even if a patient and/or family wants the provider to participate.

Not all cases, however, allow for the identification of an appropriate decision maker. Where the appropriate decision maker cannot be identified, the involved parties should have recourse to established and fair mechanisms for resolving the dispute. This may include institutional procedures for dispute resolution, such as utilizing the social work department to seek a state appointed guardian, or it may mean convening a quality review board in cases of alleged professional misconduct. As a last resort, involved parties may turn to the courts.

What are the goals of health care ethics consultation?

The general goal of health care ethics consultation is to:

- improve the provision of health care and its outcome through the identification, analysis and resolution of ethical issues as they emerge in clinical cases in health care institutions.

This general goal is more likely to be achieved if consultation accomplishes the intermediary goals of helping to:

- identify and analyze the nature of the value uncertainty or conflict that underlies the consultation
- facilitate resolution of conflicts in a respectful atmosphere with attention to the interests, rights, and responsibilities of those involved.[13]

Successful health care ethics consultation will also serve the goal of helping to:

- inform institutional efforts at policy development, quality improvement, and appropriate utilization of resources by identifying the causes of ethical problems and promoting practices consistent with ethical norms and standards[14]
- assist individuals in handling current and future ethical problems by providing education in health care ethics.[15]

1.2 The Process of Ethics Consultation

The process of ethics consultation, broadly construed, starts with a request for consultation and concludes with an evaluation. This process raises complex and often controversial moral and political questions as well as simple practical ones. Though the central focus of this report is the core competencies for doing ethics consultation discussed in section 2 below, we think it is important to address the following normative questions concerning the process of ethics consultation:

- Who should have access to ethics consultation services?
- Should patients be notified if a consult is called?

- Should ethics consultations be documented?
- Must a consultation service have a mechanism for case review?

The answers to these questions have implications for how the potentially competing rights and responsibilities of patients, families, surrogates, health care providers, and health care institutions are balanced. They also will help determine whether an ethics consultation service can function effectively in particular health care institutions. In sorting through these process issues an appropriate balance must be struck between a formal, legalistic, approach that tries to fashion rigid rules to capture every case and an approach that appeals only to abstract principles that are so general that they do not give genuine guidance.

In an effort to avoid these two extremes, we offer the following guidance:

Who should have access? Patients, families, surrogates, health care providers, and other involved parties should have access to ethics consultation services. We think that a general policy of open access is an important way of ensuring that the rights and values of all involved parties are respected. Requests for ethics consultation by patients, families, or surrogates should be honored as a matter of policy. Whereas consultations requested by health care providers or others should be provided, we realize that reasonable people may disagree about whether these consultations may be limited (for example, whether it is appropriate for an attending physician to limit consultants' direct access to patients or surrogates). Exceptions to a general policy of open access should be carefully considered and clearly delineated in the institution's ethics consultation policy.

Should patients be notified? Patients or their surrogates (in cases of incompetent patients) should be notified that an ethics consultation has been called in situations where their participation in decision making is ethically required. Notification means giving the reason for the consultation, describing the process of ethics consultation, and inviting the patient to participate as desired. The attending physician should also be notified when patient involvement is ethically required because the attending is ultimately responsible for patient care. Anyone (patient, surrogate, family, or health care provider) can refuse to participate in an ethics consultation, although a refusal is often a sign of a serious breakdown in communication and trust. Whether ethics consultations may go forward when patients refuse to participate is more controversial. In some cases, consultants may be able to help health care providers think through the ethical dimensions of the case even when patients (or other involved parties) refuse to participate. In these cases, confidentiality should be respected in a way that is consistent with consultation achieving this goal (e.g., names or other specific identifiers could be omitted).

There are consults that do not automatically demand patient involvement, such as a consult called to resolve a dispute between two health care providers or to provide information. Suppose a provider requests clarification concerning the informed consent policy or requests help resolving a question concerning conscientious objection to participation in a procedure. Exceptions to the guideline that patients should be notified that a consultation has been called should be clearly spelled out in the consultation service's policies. What should be avoided in all cases is a weakening or usurpation of legitimate decision-making authority, whether it is that of patients or health care providers.

Documentation. Ethics consultations should be documented either in the patient record, or in some other permanent record. The results of consultations ethically requiring patient involvement should be communicated to patients. All consultation services should have a policy specifying the degree and type of documentation required for consults. Such documentation promotes accountability, optimizes communication, and facilitates quality improvement.

Case review. Ethics consultation services should have a mechanism for case review to promote accountability. This process will also promote one of the goals of ethics consultation outlined above: to inform institutional efforts at policy development, quality improvement, and appropriate utilization of resources. If consultations are provided by individuals, retrospective review of those consultations by a full committee could serve this purpose. More formal evaluation methods could also serve this goal (see section 4).

Finally, it is important that each consult service clearly specify its procedures, justify them, and periodically reevaluate how they are meeting overall service and institutional objectives and values.

2. Core Competencies for Health Care Ethics Consultation

2.1 Core Competencies: The Rationale

The ultimate concern of this Task Force is quality improvement in ethics consultation. Patients, families, surrogates, and health care providers deserve assurance that when they seek help sorting through the ethical dimensions of health care, ethics consultants are competent to offer that assistance. Given the nature and goals of ethics consultation as we have described them above, we believe consultants must possess certain skills, knowledge, and character traits to perform competently. We begin by identifying these core competencies and looking at how they could be distributed among individuals, teams, and committees. Then we highlight a variety of ways individuals or groups might acquire these core competencies. Some involve formal education or training whereas others involve less traditional means such as self-study or first-hand experience. The latter were especially important for those doing consultation before adequate formal educational and training opportunities were available. Indeed, we recognize that many of those who have worked in the field for a long period of time have acquired the requisite competencies.

We also do not claim that our discussion of ways of acquiring core competencies is exhaustive nor do we believe that any particular way of acquiring a given competency should be preferred. What is important is that ethics consultants have the competencies it requires. The supplemental education or training that any individual may need to acquire a particular competency will be contingent upon at least two factors: (1) their professional background, experience, and personal qualities and (2) the capacity in which they do ethics consultation, whether as an individual consultant, as part of a consultation team, or as part of a full ethics committee.

In this report, we do not take a position on whether ethics consultation is best done by individuals, teams, or committees. Each method has certain strengths and weaknesses. The committee method, though cumbersome, has the strength of involving a wider variety of perspectives. The individual method, while lacking the variety of perspectives afforded by a committee, is well suited to bedside consultation. The team method exhibits to a lesser degree each of these strengths and weaknesses.

Individual consultants. Where ethics consultation is offered by an individual consultant, the consultant should have all of the core competencies required for ethics consultation (see sections 2.2 and 2.3). This will vary from individual to individual as each brings different strengths to ethics consultation based on their professional backgrounds, life experience, and personal qualities. Ethics consultants normally will need to supplement their professional backgrounds in order to complement the competencies that they already possess. For example:

- Clinicians might have to supplement their professional strengths to acquire advanced knowledge of moral reasoning and skill in ethical analysis, advanced knowledge of bioethical issues and concepts, basic knowledge of ethics-related health law, and advanced skill in building moral consensus.
- Lawyers with expertise in ethics-related health law might need to acquire basic knowledge of the clinical context, advanced knowledge of moral reasoning and skill in ethical analysis, advanced knowledge of common concepts and issues in bioethics, and advanced skill in resolving moral uncertainty or conflict.
- Philosophers with a specialization in ethics may need to acquire basic knowledge of the clinical context, advanced skill in enabling various parties to communicate effectively and to be heard by others, advanced listening and communication skills, basic knowledge of ethics-related health law, and various other skills and knowledge identified by this Task Force.[16]

Consultation teams. In a consultation team, the team should embody the full range of core competencies required for ethics consultation as identified in sections 2.2 and 2.3 below. Since these core competencies will be distributed among the team, less of a demand is placed on any individual team member. Depending on the team's composition, individuals may need training so that the team has the full range of competencies. Using the above example, suppose a consultation team included a philosopher, a lawyer, and a clinician. In this case, team members may need to obtain additional group process and interpersonal skills, advanced knowledge of the health care organization's relevant policies, and other skills or knowledge as needed.

Although there are certain core competencies that need only be possessed by one or more members of the team, there is certain basic knowledge and skill that every member of the team should possess. This is needed because of small group dynamics and the importance of each team member being able to fully participate in case discussions. Thus, in addition to what the group collectively must embody, each consultation team member should take steps to acquire the basic competencies outlined in Tables 1 and 2 under the heading "Every Team Member Needs."

Ethics committees. A great strength of ethics committees is that they typically are multidisciplinary. Like consultation teams, the ethics committee should collectively have the full range of core competencies for ethics consultation. Since core competencies in ethics committees will be distributed over a larger number of people, the demand placed on any particular member is less than for consultation teams, and far less than for individual consultants.

Because a committee, like a consultation team, is more than the sum of its parts, it is important that each member have certain basic skills and knowledge for addressing the types of issues that often come before it. This is especially important for enabling different viewpoints to be heard in the committee's discussion. In addition to the core competencies that the group must collectively possess, every ethics committee member should have the basic competencies listed in Tables 1 and 2 under the heading "Every Committee Member Needs."

2.2 Core Skills for Ethics Consultation

We believe that ethics consultation requires three categories of skills: (1) ethical assessment skills, (2) process skills, and (3) interpersonal skills. We distinguish between "basic" and "advanced" skill in each of these categories. For the purposes of this work, basic skill is defined as the ability to use the skill in common and straightforward cases. Advanced skill is defined as the ability to use the skill effectively in more complex cases. The distinction between basic and advanced skill is necessarily vague and somewhat arbitrary. Those with advanced skill could have either a more highly developed skill to handle more difficult cases or more complex skills. In patient interviewing, for example, being able to take a history is considered a basic skill, while attending to an anxious patient's affect while taking a history or negotiating treatment options with patients who abuse drugs are considered more advanced skills. The purpose of the distinction is to provide general guidance regarding the type and level of skills required for ethics consultation, leaving the task of more detailed operational definitions to those who provide educational and training opportunities.

Ethical assessment skills. In order to identify the nature of the value uncertainty or conflict that underlies the need for consultation, the consultant should have the ability to:

- discern and gather relevant data (e.g., clinical, psychosocial)
- assess the social and interpersonal dynamics of the case (e.g., power relations, racial, ethnic, cultural, and religious differences)
- distinguish the ethical dimensions of the case from other, often overlapping, dimensions (e.g., legal, medical, psychiatric)
- identify various assumptions that involved parties bring to the case (e.g., regarding quality of life, risk taking, unarticulated agendas)
- identify relevant values of involved parties.

Among the skills necessary to analyze the value uncertainty or conflict, the consultant must have the ability to:

- access the relevant knowledge (e.g., bioethics, law, institutional policy, professional codes, and religious teachings)
- clarify relevant concepts (e.g., confidentiality, privacy, informed consent, best interest)
- critically evaluate and use relevant knowledge of bioethics, law (without giving legal advice), institutional policy (e.g., guidelines on withdrawing or withholding life-sustaining treatment), and professional codes in the case.

To critically evaluate and use relevant knowledge, the consultant must also have the ability to:

- utilize relevant moral considerations in helping to analyze the case
- identify and justify a range of morally acceptable options and their consequences
- evaluate evidence and arguments for and against different options
- recognize and acknowledge personal limitations and possible areas of conflict between personal moral views and one's role in doing consultation (e.g., this may involve accepting group decisions with which one disagrees, but which are morally acceptable).

To acquire basic skill in ethical assessment, one needs training and experience in identifying and analyzing ethical issues. This can be acquired through: bioethics intensive courses; conferences and seminars in bioethics; bioethics presentations or in-services at one's local institution; traditional academic courses in bioethics, ethics, or moral theology; structured mentoring processes or independent studies; self-education; or educational programs that are offered by regional bioethics networks.[17]

To acquire advanced ethical assessment skills, one normally needs a longer period of education and training. Some ways of acquiring advanced ethical assessment skills include: fellowship programs that have significant emphasis on developing such skills in the clinical setting; some regional bioethics programs that have developed more advanced courses and seminars in this area; structured clinical practicums or mentoring processes that emphasize skills of ethical assessment in actual case consults; and advanced academic programs in ethics, bioethics, or medical humanities—provided they have significant emphasis on ethical analysis.[18]

In addition to programs in bioethics, other academic programs, such as those in philosophy and theology or religious studies, have traditionally offered specialized courses in ethical analysis. A series of individual courses or the completion of degree requirements in these programs is likely to provide advanced skills of ethical assessment for these purposes.

It should be noted that skills of ethical assessment in ethics consultation involve the identification and analysis of ethical issues that emerge in particular clinical cases. In these programs, case-based teaching is important. For the purposes of ethics consultation, identifying and analyzing the ethical dimensions of actual cases as they emerge in clinical settings provides a critical supplement, or even alternative, to classroom-based approaches. Conversely, clinically based approaches need to provide the knowledge (see section 2.2 below) and analytical tools traditionally imparted through classroom-based approaches.

Process skills. Though also important for ethical assessment, process skills focus on efforts to resolve the value uncertainty or conflict as it emerges in health care settings.

Process skills include the ability to facilitate formal and informal meetings. Ethics consultants must be able to:

- identify key decision-makers and involved parties and include them in discussion
- set ground rules for formal meetings (e.g., the length, participants, purpose, and structure of such meetings)
- express and stay within the limits of ethics consultants' role during the meeting
- create an atmosphere of trust that respects privacy and confidentiality and that allows parties to feel free to express their concerns (e.g., skill in addressing anger, suspicion, fear or resentment; skill in addressing intimidation and disruption due to power and/or role differentials).

Process skills also include the ability to build moral consensus. Ethics consultants must be able to:

- help individuals critically analyze the values underlying their assumptions, their decision, and the possible consequences of that decision
- negotiate between competing moral views
- engage in creative problem solving.

Process skills likewise require the ability to utilize institutional structures and resources to facilitate the implementation of the chosen option.

Lastly, process skills demand the ability to document consults and elicit feedback regarding the process of consultation so that the process can be evaluated.

Interpersonal skills. Interpersonal skills are critical to nearly every aspect of ethics consultation in individual patient cases. Interpersonal skills include the ability to:

- listen well and to communicate interest, respect, support, and empathy to involved parties[19]
- educate involved parties regarding the ethical dimensions of the case
- elicit the moral views of involved parties
- represent the views of involved parties to others
- enable involved parties to communicate effectively and be heard by other parties
- recognize and attend to various relational barriers to communication.[20]

Process and interpersonal skills are acquired primarily by "doing." There is no substitute for the role of experience in their development. One may be able to discuss how to facilitate a formal meeting, for example, but until one actually gains experience in facilitating formal meetings, one will not adequately develop the skill.

Basic interpersonal and process skills should be engendered through educational and training opportunities that are interactive and experientially based. Presentations and in-service sessions at one's local institution which include role-playing a case consultation, or running a simulated meeting would be good ways to begin to acquire basic process and interpersonal skills. Short intensive courses focused on developing these skills should also be adequate. Course work in interpersonal communication, psychology, sociology, education, or social work, provided that it includes significant interactive components, should engender basic skill in these areas as well.

The acquisition of advanced interpersonal and process skills will typically require a longer period of development and greater experience using these skills in ethics consultations. Advanced skill in these areas should equip one to handle more complex situations such as dealing with angry or confused family members or patients,

TABLE 1. Skills for Ethics Consultation

Skill Area	Individual/At Least One Member of the Group Needs	Every Team Member Needs	Every Committee Member Needs
1. Skills necessary to identify the nature of the value uncertainty or conflict that underlies the need for ethics consultation	Advanced	Basic	Basic
2. Skills necessary to analyze the value uncertainty or conflict	Advanced	Basic	Basic
3. The ability to facilitate formal and informal meetings	Advanced	Basic	Basic
4. The ability to build moral consensus	Advanced	Basic	Basic
5. The ability to utilize institutional structures and resources to facilitate the implementation of the chosen option	Basic	Not Required	Not Required
6. The ability to document consults and elicit feedback regarding the process of consultation so that the process can be evaluated	Basic	Not Required	Not Required
7. The ability to listen well and to communicate interest, respect, support, and empathy to involved parties	Advanced	Basic	Basic
8. The ability to educate involved parties regarding the ethical dimensions of the case	Basic	Not Required	Not Required
9. The ability to elicit the moral views of involved parties	Advanced	Basic	Basic
10. The ability to represent the views of involved parties to others	Advanced	Basic	Basic
11. The ability to enable the involved parties to communicate effectively and be heard by other parties	Advanced	Basic	Basic
12. The ability to recognize and attend to various relational barriers to communication	Basic	Basic	Basic

or hostile or unwilling health care professionals. As mentioned above, the development of these skills is tied to hands-on experience. Formal training in specific techniques such as mediation, conflict resolution, or facilitation is one way to obtain advanced interpersonal and process skills. Other ways of obtaining these skills include supervised clinical practicums, mentoring processes (apprenticeships with effective modeling), or fellowship programs that emphasize developing process and interpersonal skills in ethics consultation. Programs in bioethics, medical humanities and other programs such as those in the social and behavioral sciences may engender advanced skill in these areas provided they include significant and relevant experiential components.

Ethics consultants must have a variety of "basic" skills, which are used in straightforward cases, and "advanced" skills, which may be required in more complex cases. An individual ethics consultant would be expected to possess all of the skills. Every member of an ethics consultation team or committee need not have all the skills so long as they are distributed among the group.

2.3 Core Knowledge for Ethics Consultation

In addition to the skills delineated above, we believe that the nine knowledge areas indicated below are required for ethics consultation. These nine general knowledge areas overlap, and the list of subheadings will need to be revised over time due to advances in technology or changes in health care practice. In the bulleted lists, we highlight those areas that are important for ethics consultation in most institutions and so might be covered in training programs. We are aware, however, that specific issues (e.g., organ transplantation) may arise frequently in some institutions and not at all in others.

We distinguish between "basic" and "advanced" knowledge and between knowledge that should be "brought to the process" as opposed to being merely "available to the process." These terms are defined as follows: Basic knowledge is a general, or introductory, familiarity with the area specified. Advanced knowledge is a detailed grasp of the area specified. Brought to the process means that the individual(s) identified must have the knowledge to the level specified. Available to the process means that the individual consultant or at least one member of the group must know how to access advanced knowledge in the area indicated. All consultants should be aware of their own limitations and seek out specialized knowledge when appropriate.

As with the distinction between basic and advanced skill, the distinction between basic and advanced knowledge is necessarily vague and somewhat arbitrary. Again, our purpose is to provide general guidance regarding the type and level of knowledge required for ethics consultation, while leaving the detailed fleshing out to those who provide educational and training opportunities designed to instill that knowledge. Below we consider in turn (1) the knowledge area and (2) how advanced or basic knowledge might be acquired (or be available to the process where relevant).

Table 2 lists the level of knowledge in each area that individual consultants or at least one member of a team or committee needs, the knowledge that every team member needs, the knowledge that every committee member ought to have in the relevant area, and the knowledge that an individual or at least one member of a team or committee must know how to access.

Moral reasoning and ethical theory. Knowledge of moral reasoning and ethical theory should include:

- consequentialist and non-consequentialist approaches, including utilitarian, deontological approaches such as Kantian, natural law, rights theories; theological/religious approaches; and virtue, narrative, literary, and feminist approaches
- principle-based reasoning and casuistic (case-based) approaches
- related theories of justice, with particular attention to their relevance to resource allocation, triage, and rights to health care.

For ways to acquire basic and advanced knowledge in this area see the discussion following the section below.

Common bioethical issues and concepts. Knowledge of common bioethical issues and concepts includes:

- patient's rights, including rights to health care, self-determination, treatment refusal, and privacy; the concept of "positive" and "negative" rights
- autonomy and informed consent and their relation to adequate information, voluntary and involuntary, competence or decision-making capacity, rationality, paternalism
- confidentiality, including the notion of the "fiduciary" relationship of provider and patient, exceptions to confidentiality, the duty to warn, and the right to privacy
- disclosure and deception, and its relation to patients' rights, and confidentiality
- provider rights and duties, including the right to conscientious objection and the duty to care
- advance care planning, including advance directives, such as living will or durable power of attorney, and health care proxy appointments
- surrogate decision making, including decision making involving children or incapacitated/incompetent adults
- end-of-life decision making, including an understanding of do-not-resuscitate orders, withdrawal of life support, withholding nutrition and hydration; concepts of "futility," "death," "person," "quality of life," euthanasia (including the concepts of "voluntary," "involuntary," "active," and "passive euthanasia"), physician-assisted suicide and the principle of "double effect"

- beginning-of-life decision making, including reproductive technologies, surrogate parenthood, *in vitro* fertilization, sterilization, and abortion; the concept of "person," the right to privacy, and the principle of "double effect"
- genetic testing and counseling, including its relation to informed consent, paternalism, confidentiality, access to insurance, and reproductive issues
- conflicts of interest involving health care organizations, providers, and/or patients
- medical research, therapeutic innovation, or experimental treatment, and related issues of informed consent, benefit to patient, benefit to society, and social responsibility
- organ donation and transplantation, including procurement, listing of candidates, and distribution
- resource allocation, including triage, rationing, and social responsibility or obligations to society.

There are many different ways that one might come to have basic knowledge of moral reasoning and ethical theory, and issues and concepts in bioethics. These include: regional bioethics education programs, intensive courses (usually one-week courses), participation in conferences, in-service presentations, seminar sessions, and self-education. Other venues that should be sufficient to give one this basic knowledge include introductory academic courses and independent study in bioethics, ethics, or moral theology specifically tailored to these areas.

Advanced knowledge of moral reasoning/ethical theory and issues/concepts in bioethics for the purposes of ethics consultation could be acquired through: fellowship programs in ethics, moral theology, and bioethics, or an academic course or series of courses designed to give one a detailed grasp of these areas. In addition, some regional bioethics networks offer non-degree educational opportunities designed to give advanced knowledge of issues and concepts in bioethics. Some of these may have significant moral reasoning and ethical theory components as well. The completion of MA or PhD programs in bioethics, philosophy, theology, or medical humanities should be sufficient to give individuals advanced knowledge in these areas—provided that the programs have significant components in both of these knowledge areas.

Health care systems. Knowledge of health care systems includes:

- managed care systems
- governmental systems.

The vast majority of those working in health care contexts will be able to acquire basic knowledge through their work experience. For those who do not spend much time working in a health care context (e.g., some community representatives, clergy, those whose primary work is in the humanities), an introductory course in health administration or self-education should provide basic knowledge in this area.

The individual consultant or at least one member of the group must know how to access advanced knowledge in this area when necessary for the purposes of consultation in a particular case. Ethics consultants will need to have access to individuals who have extensive education and/or experience in health care systems. These persons might include officers in the institution or system or individuals with degrees in health administration.

Clinical context. Knowledge of the clinical context includes:

- terms for basic human anatomy and those used in diagnosis, treatment, and prognosis for common medical problems
- various understandings of "health" and "disease" (primarily their value-laden and socially constructed dimensions)
- awareness of the natural history of common illnesses
- awareness of the grieving process and psychological responses to illness
- awareness of the process that health care providers employ to evaluate and identify illnesses
- familiarity with current and emerging technologies that affect health care decisions
- knowledge of different health care providers, their roles, relationships, and expertise
- basic understanding of how care is provided on various services such as intensive care, rehabilitation, long-term care, palliative and hospice care, primary care, and emergency trauma care.

Health care providers will bring with them a detailed grasp of the clinical context. Clinical practicums, self-education, and introductory courses in clinical context should help others to acquire basic familiarity with clinical contexts. In-services, seminars, and conferences designed to introduce non–health care providers to the clinical context will also help individuals to acquire this knowledge.

Ethics consultants should have access to physicians, nurses, and other health care providers who have the advanced knowledge that might be needed in particular cases.

The local health care institution. Knowledge of the local health care institution includes knowing the institution's:

- mission statement
- structure, including departmental, organizational, and committee structure
- range of services and sites of delivery, such as outpatient clinic sites

- ethics consultation resources, including financial, legal, risk management, human resources, chaplain, and patient representatives
- medical research, including the role of the institutional review board, and distinctions between medical research and therapeutic innovation
- medical records, including location and access to patient records.

There is considerable overlap between this area and knowledge of health care systems. The emphasis here is on the local institution. Nearly all those who work in health care contexts will easily be able to acquire basic knowledge of their local health care institution through their professional experience. Basic familiarity in this area could also be acquired through reading the institution's policies and procedures manual or as part of a mandatory orientation session for those who work in the institution.

For advanced knowledge in this area to be available to the process of consultation, health care ethics consultants should know who in the institution to call on should detailed knowledge of some aspect of the institution be needed.

The local health care institution's policies. Knowledge of the local health care institution's policies includes understanding the facility's policies on:

- informed consent
- withholding and withdrawing life-sustaining treatment
- euthanasia (and assisted suicide, if relevant)
- advance directives, surrogate decision making, health care agents, durable power of attorney, and guardianship
- do-not-resuscitate orders
- medical futility
- confidentiality and privacy
- organ donation and procurement
- human experimentation
- conflicts of interest
- admissions, discharge and transfer
- impaired providers
- conscientious objection
- reproductive technology.

For basic knowledge, ethics consultants should be aware of the institution's relevant policies and have a general understanding of their content. One could acquire basic knowledge by reading the policies or through orientation sessions regarding the policies.

An individual should be able to acquire advanced knowledge relevant to these policies through self-education. In-service or seminar sessions on relevant policies could also promote advanced knowledge of relevant policies.

Beliefs and perspectives of local patient and staff population. Knowledge of the beliefs and perspectives of the local patient and staff population includes:

- important beliefs and perspectives that bear on the health care of racial, ethnic, cultural and religious groups served by the facility
- resource persons for understanding and interpreting cultural and faith communities.

The multicultural nature of health care institutions and the patients they serve make knowledge of different cultures and faith communities critical for consultation. Basic knowledge in this area can be acquired through in-service presentations, conferences, and seminars germane to the cultural backgrounds of patient and staff at the local institution.

Ethics consultants should have access to individuals who will have advanced knowledge of the beliefs and perspectives of various members of the patient and staff population. These individuals might include chaplains, social workers, patient representatives, mental health professionals, risk managers, sociologists, and anthropologists.

Relevant codes of ethics and professional conduct and guidelines of accrediting organizations. Knowledge of the relevant codes of ethics and professional conduct and guidelines of accrediting organizations includes:

- codes of conduct from relevant professional organizations (e.g., medicine, nursing)
- local health care facility's code of professional conduct
- other important professional and consensus ethics guidelines and statements (e.g., presidential commission statements)
- patient's bill of rights and responsibilities
- relevant standards of the JCAHO and other accrediting bodies (e.g., patient rights and organizational ethics standards).

For basic knowledge in this area, one should read the relevant code or manual.

In order for advanced knowledge in this area to be available to the process of consultation, ethics consultants should know who the contact persons might be to discuss the area in question (e.g., the person or persons responsible for the JCAHO survey). They should also know where to find the code or accreditation manual.

Relevant health law. Knowledge of relevant health law (both federal and state constitutional, statutory and case law) includes law governing:

- end-of-life issues such as advance directives (including living wills and proxy appointment documents such as durable powers of attorney), nutrition and hydration, determination of death
- surrogate decision making, including determination of incompetence, appointment of surrogates, and use of proxy appointment documents
- decision making for incompetent patients without family, intimates, or other identifiable surrogates, including medical guardianship and other mechanisms
- decision making for minors, including the need for minors' assent, minors' capacity to consent, and decision making when minors cannot consent
- informed consent
- reproductive issues
- organ donation and procurement
- confidentially, privacy, and release of information
- reporting requirements, including child, spouse, or elder abuse and communicable diseases.

Many of the means to acquire basic knowledge in bioethics as outlined above would also be helpful to acquire basic knowledge of relevant health law. These include: basic courses in health law designed to give an introduction for nonspecialists; independent study courses; regional ethics education programs that give attention to health law; intensive courses (usually one-week or weekend courses) that have health law components; participation in ongoing conferences, in-service presentations, and seminar sessions on health law; and self-education in health law.

Advanced knowledge of relevant health law would be available to the process, if ethics consultants know how to reach legal counsel with expertise in ethics-related health law.

Health care ethics consultants require "basic" introductory-level knowledge in some areas and more "advanced" detailed understanding of topics in others. We distinguish between knowledge that individuals or team members must bring to the consultation process ("needs") and knowledge that individuals or team members must have available to the consultation process ("can access"). All consultants should be aware of their limitations so that they know when they need to seek out those who might have specialized knowledge.

2.4 Character and Ethics Consultation

In addition to the core competencies considered above, all members of the Task Force agree that good character is important for optimal ethics consultation. The rationale for this belief, and opinions about the specific relationship between character and ethics consultation, depend upon a number of issues over which there is

TABLE 2. Knowledge for Ethics Consultation

Knowledge Area	Individual/ At Least One Member Needs	Every Team Member Needs	Every Committee Member Needs	Individual/ At Least One Member Can Access
1. Moral reasoning and ethical theory as it relates to ethics consultation	Advanced	Basic	Basic	Not Required
2. Bioethical issues and concepts that typically emerge in ethics consultation	Advanced	Basic	Basic	Not Required
3. Health care systems as they relate to ethics consultation	Basic	Basic	Basic	Advanced
4. Clinical context as it relates to ethics consultation	Basic	Basic	Basic	Advanced
5. Health care institution in which the consultants work, as it relates to ethics consultation	Basic	Basic	Basic	Advanced
6. Local health care institution's policies relevant for ethics consultation	Advanced	Basic	Basic	Not Required
7. Beliefs and perspectives of patient and staff population where one does ethics consultation	Basic	Basic	Basic	Advanced
8. Relevant codes of ethics, professional conduct and guidelines of accrediting organizations as they relate to ethics consultation	Basic	Not Required	Not Required	Advanced
9. Health law relevant to ethics consultation	Basic	Basic	Basic	Advanced

controversy among Task Force members. This stems, at least in part, from the close connection between character and conceptions of "the good." When people disagree about conceptions of the good, they are also likely to hold divergent conceptions of character.

In Task Force discussions of character, controversy emerged over whether:

- character is a set of observable behaviors, an internalized inclination to behave in a certain way, or a more fundamental constituent of persons
- certain traits of character are necessary for, or incidental to, the acquisition of certain kinds of skills or knowledge that may be important for various activities
- behavior can be compartmentalized so that bad behavior in one domain does not mean that it will be exhibited in other domains
- the better measure of character involves day-to-day activities or extreme tests such as those times when one must take a stand at considerable personal risk
- evaluations of bioethics consultation or consultants need to focus on more than behavior
- character traits can be correctly defined.

Although the ethics literature historically has included discussions of character, there is little contemporary study of the relationship between character and ethics consultation. This explains, in part, why the Task Force did not attempt to outline a definitive list of character traits that are necessary for ethics consultation. Instead, the Task Force offers the following points and illustrative examples to help advance the dialogue.

By pointing to a connection between character and ethics consultation and including examples, the Task Force does not suggest that all ethics consultants, including Task Force members, possess all of these traits. Also, we do not suggest that character is less important for persons in medicine, nursing, teaching, social work, pastoral care, and other professions or occupations. Nor do we suggest that ethics consultants have or must have better character than others. Nonetheless, the more a consultant possesses and exhibits certain character traits, the more likely the consultation will be effective.[21]

Traits associated with successful consultations. Below are examples of character traits or personal qualities that are believed to be related to success in ethics consultation. It should be noted that character traits cannot be divided into basic and advanced levels. The acquisition and nurturing of character is something persons should strive for over a lifetime. We conclude that all ethics consultants should strive to possess and exhibit these traits:

- *Tolerance, patience, and compassion* are traits that would enable the consultant to "listen well and communicate interest, respect, support and empathy" (skill

7, Table 1). Tolerance and patience help welcome people with difficult problems, those who may be emotionally distraught, or those who have minority views, so that these people can be fully and respectfully heard. Compassion helps the consultant to work constructively with feelings in sometimes tragic situations.

• *Honesty, forthrightness and self-knowledge* are traits that will help prevent the manipulative use of information and help "create an atmosphere of trust" necessary to facilitate formal and informal meetings (skill 3, Table 1). Consultants must be honest about their own limitations, their need for more knowledge, how their agendas and values are shaping the consultation, and the uncertainty about proposed solutions.

• *Courage* is sometimes needed to enable various parties, especially the politically less powerful, to communicate effectively and be heard by other parties (skill 11, Table 1). It is also sometimes required to take positions that are unpopular or contrary to the interests of one's employer or other powerful individuals.

• *Prudence and humility* can inform behavior when rash or novel courses of action are being considered and enable consultants not to overstep the bounds of their role in consultation. These character traits can help consultants acknowledge possible areas of conflict between their personal moral views and their role in doing consultation (skill 4, Table 1).

• *Integrity* would enable consultants to pursue the option or range of options ethically required in the case even when it might be convenient to do otherwise (skill 5, Table 1). Integrity should inform all behavior of consultants as they strive to fulfill the trust placed in them by health care providers, patients, and families who seek help resolving ethical issues.

Good character, and integrity in particular, is not only important for conducting ethics consultation itself, but also for the credibility of those who will be conducting it. Other professionals and lay persons understandably expect that good character be exhibited by ethics consultants in their professional roles (and indeed in other quasi-public domains). The perception of a person's character in these other areas will inevitably influence one's effectiveness in doing a consult. For example, a physician who developed a reputation for belittling other members of the health care team or routinely disregarding the wishes of competent patients would face a serious credibility problem in performing ethics consultations.

Nurturing character. Most Task Force members also agree that character can be nurtured and that its importance for ethics consultation should be taught and modeled. All Task Force members agree that the controversies surrounding character and consultation identified above need to be acknowledged and discussed as well.

Programs to educate persons for health care ethics consultation should at least:

• encourage reflection about character and its development and explore the possible relationship between character and clinical ethics consultation
• use faculty or mentors who model these important traits of character and who are willing to reflect with students on whether and how character contributed to past successful or unsuccessful consultations
• hold consultants in training accountable for their behavior.

3. Organizational Ethics

3.1 Defining Organizational Ethics

Organizational ethics deals with an organization's positions and behavior relative to individuals (including patients, providers, and employees), groups, communities served by the organization, and other organizations.[22] These positions and behavior may be reflected, for example, in explicit or implicit mission and vision statements, policies, procedures, contracts, agreements, and public and private communications and actions. Ethical issues in organizational behavior have become more evident in recent years with the emergence of a more explicit market approach to medicine. Areas in which value conflict or uncertainty have arisen include billing practices, access to health care, financial incentives for clinicians, restrictions on access to specialists, and marketing. Some examples of organizational ethics consultations follow:

• A financial officer informally requests advice from an ethics consultant in resolving his uncertainty over the development of a procedure for "unbundling" services for billing purposes in order to increase revenue.
• A health plan medical director requests assistance from an ethics consultation service in negotiating a conflict between the plan's CEO and the plan's physicians over a proposed financial incentive program for clinicians.
• A physician formally requests intervention by a bioethics committee in resolving a conflict with the medical director over whether her patient should receive an experimental therapy not covered by the patient's insurance.

As these examples demonstrate, the resolution of many value conflicts and uncertainties in organizational ethics either requires consideration of values historically considered within the domain of clinical ethics and/or have ramifications for the clinical care of individual patients.

Many of these issues and their potential for conflict have existed for years, but were largely hidden or ignored because of the traditional separation of the functions of providing individual care, improving population health, and financing health care. Practitioners in each area have developed their own ethical traditions and boundaries. Thus, potential conflicts in decision making that stem from differences in these traditions and boundaries—especially between the traditions of clinical ethics and of business ethics—were typically not the subject of bioethics consultation. The intersection between the bedside, community, and boardroom, has become inescapable, however, as the delivery and financing of health care have been increasingly centralized in health care systems and as cost containment has become a national concern. Increasingly, value conflicts and uncertainties cross these three ethical domains, and their resolution can now affect behavior and outcomes in all three domains.

For these reasons, the Task Force believes that no clear and absolute line can be drawn between organizational ethics and clinical ethics. Ethics consultants, then, will increasingly be unable to provide consultation services in one area while ignoring the other. It is thus useful for clinical ethics committees to encourage membership by non-clinical administrators as one way of cultivating mutual respect for and critical analysis of each other's ethical traditions.

Limitations in knowledge. Despite the important relationship between clinical and organizational ethics, the ability of the Task Force to make recommendations regarding organizational ethics consultation is limited by several factors:

• The state of knowledge about organizational ethics consultation in health care is still developing. Compared with clinical ethics consultation, there is much less descriptive literature about the types of cases encountered and the various efforts to resolve them through consultation.

• The collective education/experience of Task Force members in clinical ethics consultation far outweighs their education/experience in organizational ethics.

• The type of assistance being sought by individuals who request organizational ethics consultation and how those experienced in clinical ethics consultation might be helpful is less well established.

Differences between clinical and organizational ethics. It is also important to bear in mind some differences between the two types of ethics consultation:

• The focus of a request for clinical consultation usually falls within a known list of issues, and knowledge of the basic technical content relevant to the various issues can be mastered by consultants. In organizational consultation, the rapidly changing structure and financing of health care have meant that knowledge about the technical content of the issue under consideration often has to be learned within the context of the consultation itself.

• The party that pays for the consultation in clinical consultation is generally not one of the directly involved parties. In organizational consultation, the party that pays for the consultation—the health care organization—frequently is involved directly in the decision making.

- Consultants in clinical consultation often provide consultation to others who are lateral or below them in the organizational hierarchy. In organizational consultation, those who use consultants' services are often senior leaders who in the organizational hierarchy are higher than the consultants.

- The impact of any resolution in organizational ethics consultation is wider in scope. That is, it will affect many patients, many practitioners, many employees—not just those involved in a specific case. And the impact of the resolution persists over a longer time. Both predicting and monitoring its long-term consequences may be part of the consultation process.

Similarities between clinical and organizational ethics. Though there are differences between clinical and organizational ethics consultation, the context of societal, institutional, communal, professional, and individual values that frames issues in clinical ethics also frames issues in organizational ethics. Moreover, the fundamental goal of organizational ethics consultation and clinical case consultation is the same: to help people resolve uncertainty or conflict regarding value-laden issues. The Task Force believes that the ethics-facilitation approach suggested for clinical ethics consultation may be appropriate for organizational ethics consultation. If this is true, organizational ethics consultation will require many of the same skills and knowledge needed for clinical ethics consultation.

The Task Force acknowledges, however, that the ethics-facilitation approach would need to be adapted to the different issues and concerns raised by organizational ethics, and that other approaches may also be appropriate. Because the differing traditions and boundaries of clinical ethics and business ethics are both relevant in organizational ethics consultation, a resolution based on consensus may be more difficult to achieve than in conflicts or uncertainties that fall entirely within one tradition and its set of boundaries. Moreover, it may be more difficult to identify relevant involved parties for consensus building in organizational ethics consultation. Thus, at a minimum, further exploration of various approaches to organizational ethics issues and their advantages and disadvantages is needed.

The Task Force also notes that although there is a growing emphasis on compliance programs that often address ethical issues, organizational ethics encompasses a scope much broader than the legal sphere. Some decisions that comply with the law may, nevertheless, be considered unethical.

3.2 *Some Preliminary Recommendations*

At this early stage, it appears that the most salient difference between clinical and organizational ethics consultation concerns the types of issues raised. Clinical ethics consultants will, therefore, need to obtain the additional knowledge to inform, mediate discussion of, and facilitate resolution of uncertainty or conflict regarding value-laden issues in organizational ethics. Organizational ethics consultation may require knowledge about:

- health care business, cost-containment and managed care ethics, including cost shifting, billing practices, financial or administrative incentives on clinicians, resource allocation, definitions of standard or experimental care, and conflicts of interest
- interactions with the marketplace of medicine, including the endorsement of medical products for the purposes of market promotion, and issues raised in marketing health care organizations, such as truth in advertising and promotion of unrealistic expectations
- societal and public health obligations, including serving the medically underserved, antidumping policies, culturally sensitive care, discrimination against or by patients (e.g., based on age, race, gender, sexual orientation, religion, disability, disease, or socioeconomic status), and public disclosure of measures of organizational performance or clinical errors
- scientific and educational health care, including institutional obligations in training future health care providers or in performing research
- general business issues, including relationships with employees (e.g., discrimination in hiring and promotion, conscientious objection of employees), suppliers (e.g., bidding and contracting practices), payers (e.g., cost accounting practices), regulators (e.g., political contributions), shareholders and creditors (e.g., financial reporting), and the public (e.g., conflicts of interest in roles).

Consultation regarding these types of issues will require education in areas ranging from the health care organization's business and administrative structures, the health care system's current structure, the economics of health care (including financing mechanisms and cost-benefit analysis), and the variety of business arrangements in medicine.

Given the early state in the development of organizational ethics consultation and the lack of experience in this area, we think that more detailed recommendations would be inappropriate at this time. We encourage additional efforts, including both empirical and conceptual research, to define more clearly the scope of organizational ethics consultation; the most effective and efficient organizational structures for its delivery (e.g., its relationship to existing ethics committees); the degree to which it should include preemptive, unsolicited interventions; the appropriate approaches for dealing with organizational ethics issues; and the knowledge and experience that it demands. We also recommend that managed care plans and health care organizations develop methods for identifying and addressing the organizational ethics issues they face.

4. The Importance of Evaluation

4.1 Where Is Evaluation Needed?

A full discussion of the purposes and techniques of evaluation is beyond the scope of this report. The Task Force attaches great importance to evaluation, however, and sees it as an area that should be actively pursued through research and practice. Evaluation of ethics consultation is needed in three areas: the competencies of those who do ethics consultation, the process of consultation itself, and the outcomes of consultation.

Evaluating consultants. It is important to assess the degree to which individuals have the core competencies described above. This is especially critical for programs that train individuals to do ethics consultation. To the extent that educators are persuaded that these competencies are important for ethics consultation, they should take steps to ensure that their educational objectives cover these competencies and that they have reliable measures for identifying whether those objectives are achieved. For many of the process and interpersonal skills identified above, traditional testing methods, such as essay, short-answer, or multiple choice, may be unreliable. Observing someone perform a consultation (or a "mock" consultation), for example, will be a better way of assessing facilitation skills than evaluating an essay about how to do a consultation.

Evaluating the process. Evaluation of the consultation process is needed. Above we addressed several important normative questions raised by the process of consultation. We recommended that every ethics consultation service have clearly specified procedures for consultation that are consistent with the position that the Task Force took on those normative questions. Evaluation is important for determining whether the procedures of a consult service are being followed. Chart reviews, for example, could indicate whether consults are properly documented or patient/ family surveys could help to confirm that notification procedures are being followed.

Evaluating outcomes. The outcomes of ethics consultation must also be evaluated. This is both the most important and most difficult evaluation area. Evaluating outcomes is an important way to justify and correct recommended competencies for consultants and process procedures. No reliable data, for example, is currently available demonstrating that consultants who possess certain competencies do "better" consultations. Similarly, there is no reliable data on what methods of ethics consultation best achieve its goals. Moreover, despite the current trend toward instituting quality assurance techniques throughout health care, such efforts have been meager in ethics consultation.

One of the major impediments to evaluating ethics consultation outcomes has been the lack of specification of consultation's goals. Based on the goals delineated above, the Task Force suggests that consultation be evaluated answering the following questions:[23]

- Was a consensus reached?
- Was the consensus within the boundaries set by societal values, law, and institutional policy?
- Was the consensus implemented?
- What was the level of satisfaction among participants?[24]

It is too early to endorse specific methods, either quantitative or qualitative, for assessment of ethics consultation. A wide variety of methods should be pursued. Simple qualitative methods, which can be initiated even by consultants without a great deal of expertise in evaluation technique, remain useful. Members of an ethics committee, for example, could review consultations performed by an individual consultant, or an outside consultant could review the ethics committee's activities. These reviews should always be systematic and rigorous with careful attention to purpose and technique. They can serve the purpose of making sure that consultations follow an organization's procedural guidelines and do not result in decisions that reflect consultants' idiosyncratic views.

Quantitative evaluation of ethics consultation also could prove useful in assessing ethics consultations in each of the areas discussed above: the competencies of consultants, the process of consultation, and the outcomes of consultation. Formal quantitative evaluation can help answer questions such as whether certain consultation processes or methods (such as individuals, teams, or committees) best achieve ethics consultation's goals, whether there is a correlation between the competencies of consultants and the outcomes of ethics consultation, and whether relevant ethics policies are more likely to be adhered to in practice if an institution has ethics consultation. Quantitative evaluation requires the development of reliable, valid instruments, and careful attention to methodological issues. These assessments should be carried out by those with expertise in evaluation research or quality improvement.[25]

5. Special Obligations of Ethics Consultants and Institutions

Before concluding this report, we address two remaining areas of concern. The first involves the dangers of the abuse of power and conflict of interest by those who do ethics consultation. The second involves institutional obligations to support those who offer ethics consultation services. These two areas are related: Satisfying institutional obligations to support ethics consultation, for example, will decrease the risk that consultants themselves will abuse their position.

5.1 Abuse of Power and Conflict of Interest

By virtue of their role in health care institutions, ethics consultants are both granted and claim social authority to influence:

- the clinical care of patients
- the behavior of health care providers toward families of patients and toward each other
- the behavior of health care institutions toward patients, families, health care providers, and the larger community.

It is therefore inevitable that ethics consultants hold a certain degree of power that, under certain circumstances, can be abused. The potential for abuse of power is not unique to ethics consultants, but instead, a problem for all health care providers. It is inherent in the nature of their role and specialized knowledge, as well as the vulnerability of the persons they serve. The potential imbalance of power imposes a special obligation on ethics consultants not to abuse this power.

Many of the professional or academic backgrounds from which ethics consultants come have codes of conduct governing potential abuse of power. Not all professions and settings do, however, and existing codes are neither uniform nor do they cover the specific role of ethics consultants. For this reason, it is necessary to address some important potential abuses of power:

- Ethics consultants have access to privileged information including highly personal medical, psychological, financial, legal and spiritual data. The requirements of confidentiality must be respected.
- If ethics consultants have significant personal or professional relationships with one or more parties that could lead to bias, that relationship should be disclosed and/or the consultants should remove themselves from the case.
- Individuals should never serve as ethics consultants on cases in which they have clinical and/or administrative responsibility.
- There is a potential conflict of interest when ethics consultants are employed by a health care institution or their jobs are dependent on the good will of the institution. Giving advice or otherwise acting against the institution's perceived financial, public relations, or other interest may pose potential harm to ethics consultants' personal interests. This issue should be addressed proactively with the health care institution by any individual or group that plans to offer ethics consultation in that institution. If the conflict of interest in an individual case puts ethics consultants in the position of shading an opinion to avoid personal risk, they should either take that risk or withdraw from the case.
- Ethics consultants should never exploit those persons they serve by using their position of power. Ethics consultants, for example, should not take sexual or financial advantage of those they serve.

The above mentioned cautions should be discussed and explained thoroughly in the training of ethics consultants.

5.2 Institutional Obligations to Patients, Providers, and Consultants

The dangers of abuse of power and conflict of interest can be mitigated if health care institutions take seriously their obligations to those who provide and utilize ethics consultation services. When patients, families, surrogates, or health care providers seek assistance in sorting through the ethical dimensions of health care, they deserve assurance that those who offer that assistance are competent to do so and can offer that assistance free of undue pressure. We have discussed in detail how important it is for those who do ethics consultation to take seriously quality assurance and improvement. We have also underscored the dangers of abuse of power and conflict of interest on the part of consultants. Nonetheless, the burden of satisfying these obligations should not fall solely on the shoulders of those who offer ethics consultation. Health care institutions must be responsible to those who utilize ethics consultation services by providing support for ethics consultants in their institution. This support is needed in three areas:

• Health care institutions should support a clear process by which ethics consultants are educated, trained and appointed, and provide the resources for those who offer ethics consultation to ensure that they have the competencies to perform consultation. This will require support for continuing education and access to core bioethics resources (such as key reference texts, journals, and on-line services).

• Health care institutions should ensure that those who offer ethics consultation are given adequate time and compensation for non-remunerative activities, and resources to do ethics consultation properly.

• Health care institutions should seek to foster a climate in which those offering ethics consultation services can carry out their work with integrity (e.g., a climate free of concerns about job security, reprisals, undue political pressure). This should include separating ethics consultation from personnel oversight, so that health care providers see ethics consultation as a resource for addressing ethical uncertainties or conflicts rather than as a disciplinary action, and respecting the independence of ethics consultation and ethics policy initiatives. In such a climate, pressures to abuse power or give in to conflict of interest will be significantly diminished.

III. Using the Task Force Report

Voluntary guidelines. The Task Force unanimously recommends that the content of this report be used as voluntary guidelines. Whether these guidelines are adopted by health care organizations or education and training programs should be based on an informed discussion of the report's merits. The Task Force:

- does not wish certifying or accrediting bodies to mandate any portion of its report
- believes that certification of individuals or groups to do ethics consultation is, at best, premature
- does not intend for its report [to be] used to establish a legal national standard for competence to do ethics consultation for the reasons indicated below.

The Task Force endorses voluntary guidelines for a number of reasons. First, as voluntary guidelines, the recommendations in this report reflect the complexity and lack of data surrounding the current state of ethics consultation. Second, voluntary guidelines are sensitive to the wide diversity of institutional settings where consultation takes place (e.g., the needs of large teaching hospitals differ tremendously from those of small community hospitals or long-term care facilities). Third, although they remain tentative, voluntary guidelines can encourage gradual change and stimulate public discussion. Finally, whether voluntary guidelines are adopted depends, at least in part, on the guidelines' merit.

The alternatives to a voluntary model, certification and accreditation, have serious drawbacks that led the Task Force to reject them. The Task Force viewed these drawbacks as strong reasons to endorse the voluntary model.

The drawbacks of certification. The Task Force rejects the certification of individuals or groups to do ethics consultation for many reasons.[26] First, certification increases the risk of displacing providers and patients as the primary moral decision makers at the bedside because it can give the impression that certified individuals have special standing in ethical decision making. Certification, then, could encourage the type of authoritarian approach to ethics consultation the Task Force has rejected.

Second, certification could undermine disciplinary diversity if it fell under the control of a particular discipline and was widely adopted. The Task Force believes that this would be undesirable because the different disciplines involved in ethics consultation each bring identifiable strengths to the process. Philosophers, for example, typically bring a strong background in ethical analysis, while social workers bring excellent facilitation skills. It is important that consultants have the relevant competencies, not that they come from some particular professional or academic field. The Task Force believes that the interdisciplinary nature of the field leads to a more balanced understanding of competencies important for doing ethics consultation.

Third, certification could lead to the institutionalization of a particular substantive view of morality, a certain view of the relation between ethical theory and practice, or one conception of the relative importance of skills that are important for ethics consultation.

Fourth, if certification of individuals or groups were based on standardized testing, the tests would have to be shown to measure the competencies in question. Considering the level of uncertainty and lack of outcome data, it is unlikely at this time that a sufficiently reliable test could be developed to measure the required competencies.

Finally, certification would also require the development of a new bureaucracy to manage it, with all the attendant costs and difficulties. This raises serious political and practical difficulties that should not be undertaken without a strong justification and a compelling need.

The drawbacks of accreditation. The Task Force rejects specially accrediting educational programs that would train individuals or groups to do ethics consultation for many of the same reasons that it rejects the certification of individuals or groups to do ethics consultation. The emergence of accredited educational programs could promote the dominance of a particular moral view or technical approach, have an adverse effect on disciplinary diversity, and imply a degree of professionalization that is, in the opinion of the Task Force, premature at best. As with certification, we believe that the practical and administrative costs of accreditation are serious enough that they should not be taken on without compelling need or justification.

Thus, at this time, the Task Force recommends that its report be used only as voluntary guidelines. The specification of "at this time" does not mean that the Task Force contemplates mandatory guidelines at some later time. Rather, the specification means our assessment is based on the current state of knowledge and our recognition that this state is evolving.

One might ask whether the concerns raised about certification and accreditation might not apply equally well to voluntary guidelines. Such an objection misses the spirit of our recommendations. In surgery, we know that perfect sterility is impossible, but no one takes this as a warrant for abandoning all precautions. What we have tried to do is to provide guidance in some very uncharted waters about, among other things, the nature and goals of ethics consultation, the core competencies that are needed to do it, and how those competencies might be acquired.

Notes

1. See Appendix 1 for a complete list of the organizations that provided financial support for this project.

2. We are indebted to the Strategic Research Network on Health Care Ethics Consultation project, which was funded by the Social Sciences and Humanities Research Council of Canada, for the idea of looking at the skills, knowledge, and character traits that are important for health care ethics consultation. This project resulted in *The Health Care Ethics Consultant* (Baylis, 1994) which was made available to members of this Task Force at the outset of our project.

3. We refer to all who do ethics consultations, whether as individuals or as part of a team or committee, as "consultants" throughout this text.

4. Throughout this document we will use the terms "ethics" and "morals" (and all their variations) interchangeably. Regarding "value," we realize that there are values embedded in many different domains (e.g., law, morals, professional practices, various communities, individual conceptions of the good). We are using "value" as a general term to capture the various normative dimensions of issues that emerge in health care. Value conflict or uncertainty often arises because of competing values from these different domains (e.g., judgments of "best treatment" often differ depending on whether medical values or individual patient values are being considered). Also, we will use "health care provider" as an umbrella category to refer to all those involved in patient care (including physicians, nurse practitioners, nurses, social workers, chaplains, nurses' aides, technicians, and others).

5. These affective dimensions will sometimes involve cases in which parties seeking consultation know what ought to be done but find it very difficult to do so for either intrapersonal or interpersonal reasons. This could occur because the choice the parties face is so daunting (e.g., agreeing to have life support withdrawn from a loved one) or because they find themselves in a difficult interpersonal relationship.

6. Throughout this document "ethics consultation" should be taken as referring to both case and policy consultation.

7. These include, for example, pressures stemming from scarcity of resources and the need for cost containment.

8. Indeed, sometimes institutional policies or laws will themselves be at odds with deep societal values. Some people would argue, for example, that this was the case with abortion before it was legalized or is presently the case with physician-assisted suicide.

9. We are not claiming that anyone actually does ethics consultation in either of these two ways. Rather, we are characterizing two extreme approaches for illustrative purposes. Most approaches fall between these two extremes, but tendencies toward one or the other can be found in the literature (Aulisio, Arnold, and Youngner, 1998).

10. As with attempts to characterize nursing or medical practice, or any other activity, there is likely to be controversy at the margins. We are interested here in giving a normative characterization of the core features of ethics consultation. Also, the ethics facilitation approach will not be applicable to every type of consult. Purely informational consults, for example, will not involve facilitation between multiple parties, as in a request for clarification regarding the institutional policy on withdrawing life-sustaining treatment.

11. Some recent legal cases have raised concerns about a proper approach to ethics consultation (Fletcher and Spencer, 1997, 270–275). One case, Gilgunn v. Massachusetts General Hospital, appears to have been handled in this authoritarian manner (Capron, 1995, 24–26).

12. By "consensus" we mean agreement by all involved parties.

13. From Fletcher and Siegler, 1996, 125.

14. *Ibid.* As this goal suggests, ethics consultation provides opportunities for education, research and policy development even as it seeks to resolve ethical questions that arise in specific clinical cases.

15. *Ibid.*

16. These examples were chosen only because they make it relatively easy to see the strengths that each individual will bring in virtue of their professional background and how they will need to supplement those strengths in light of the core competencies we discuss below.

17. See Appendix 2 for a list of departments, centers, regional networks and other organizations that submitted materials to help complete this project. See also Thornton and Callahan's, 1993, report of *The Hastings Center* on bioethics education.

18. *Ibid.*

19. See Lipkin, Putnam, and Lazare, 1995, 3–19.

20. *Ibid.*

21. As mentioned above, whether character is a set of behaviors or an internalized disposition to behave was something about which the Task Force could not agree.

22. We want to thank Myra Christopher for her comments on an early version of this section. This newly emerging area has a burgeoning literature. For example, Biblo, Christopher, Johnson, and Potter, 1995; R. L. Potter, 1996; Schyve, 1996; Kotin, 1996; Renz and Eddy, 1996; Berkowitz, 1996; and Hofmann, 1996.

23. These correspond roughly to the domains identified by Fox and Arnold, 1996. For a fuller discussion of the relevance and importance of evaluation research for ethics consultation see Fox, 1996; Fox and Tulsky, 1996; Tulsky and Stocking, 1996; Tulsky and Fox, 1996. These articles resulted from the 1995 conference on Evaluation of Care Consultation in Clinical Ethics, which was supported by a grant from the Agency for Health Care Policy and Research. At the conference there was a recognition that before rigorous evaluation of ethics consultation could be done, there was a need for some consensus on its goals. The conference resulted in a consensus statement on the goals of ethics consultation (see Fletcher and Siegler, 1996).

24. Satisfaction alone is an inadequate measure of quality in ethics consultation. For example, certain individuals might be quite satisfied with what turned out to be a morally inappropriate course of action (suppose the course of action involved imposing a treatment on a competent patient against her will).

25. See, for example, Patton, 1987, or Fink, 1993.

26. Certification, for our purposes, refers to documentation by a certifying body, often through standardized testing, that an individual or group has the necessary knowledge, skills, and character to engage in a certain practice. Thus, individuals or groups who are certified can claim that they have the minimal qualifications needed for the practice. Often stronger claims are made for certification, e.g., that the uncertified should be barred from practice.

Bibliography

Ackerman, T.F. (1987). The role of an ethicist in health care. In G.R. Anderson & V.A. Glesnes-Anderson (Eds.), *Health care ethics: A guide for decision makers* (pp. 308–320). Rockville, MD: Aspen Publishers.

Ackerman, T.F. (1989). Conceptualizing the role of the ethics consultant: Some theoretical issues. In J.C. Fletcher, N. Quist, & A.R. Jonsen (Eds.), *Ethics consultation in health care* (pp. 37–52). Ann Arbor, MI: Health Administration Press.

Ackerman, T.F. (1989). Moral problems, moral inquiry, and consultation in clinical ethics. In

B. Hoffmaster, B. Freedman, & G. Fraser (Eds.), *Clinical ethics: Theory and practice* (pp. 141–160). Clifton, NJ: Humana Press.

Agich, G.J. (1990). Clinical ethics: A role theoretic look. *Social Science and Medicine, 30*, 389–399.

Agich, G.J. (1994). Expertise in clinical ethics consultation. *HEC Forum, 6*, 379–383.

Agich, G.J., & Youngner, S.J. (1991). For experts only? Access to hospital ethics committees. *Hastings Center Report, 21*(5), 17–25.

Anderson, C.A. (1996). Ethics committees and quality improvement: A necessary link. *Journal of Nursing Care Quality, 11*(1), 22–28.

Andre, J. (1997). Goals of ethics consultation: Toward clarity, utility, and fidelity. *The Journal of Clinical Ethics, 8*, 193–198.

Aulisio, M.P., Arnold, R.M., & Youngner, S.J. (1998). Can there be educational and training standards for those conducting health care ethics consultation? In D. Thomasma & J. Monagle (Eds.), *Health care ethics: Critical issues for the twenty-first century* (pp. 484–496). Gaithersburg, MD: Aspen Publishers.

Barnard, D. (1992). Reflections of a reluctant clinical ethicist: Ethics consultation and the collapse of critical distance. *Theoretical Medicine, 13*, 15–22.

Baylis, F. (1989). Persons with moral expertise and moral experts: Wherein lies the difference? In B. Hoffmaster, B. Freedman, & G. Fraser (Eds.), *Clinical ethics: Theory and practice* (pp. 89–99). Clifton, NJ: Humana Press.

Baylis, F.E. (Ed.) (1994). *The health care ethics consultant.* Totowa, NJ: Humana Press.

Baylis, F.E. (1994). A profile of the health care ethics consultant. In F.E. Baylis (Ed.), *The health care ethics consultant* (pp. 25–44). Totowa, NJ: Humana Press.

Berkowitz, E.N. (1996). The evolving health care marketplace: How important is the patient? *Bioethics Forum, 12*(2), 40–44.

Biblo, J.D., Christopher, M.J., Johnson, L., & Potter, R.L. (1995). *Ethical issues in managed care: Guidelines for clinicians and recommendations to accrediting organizations.* Kansas City, MO: Midwest Bioethics Center, Bioethics Development Group.

Browne, A., & Sweeney, V.P. (1996). Ethics committee education: A report on a Canadian project. *HEC Forum, 8*, 290–300.

Buehler, D. (1997). CQ sources/bibliography. *Cambridge Quarterly of Healthcare Ethics, 6*, 302–305.

Callahan, D. (1996). Bioethics, our crowd, and ideology. *Hastings Center Report, 26*(6), 3–4.

Caplan, A. (1989). Moral experts and moral expertise: Do either exist? In B. Hoffmaster, B. Freedman, & G. Fraser (Eds.), *Clinical ethics: Theory and practice* (pp. 59–87). Clifton, NJ: Humana Press.

Capron, A.M. (1995). Abandoning a waning life. *Hastings Center Report, 25*(4), 24–26.

Christensen, K.T., & Tucker, R. (1997). Ethics without walls: The transformation of ethics committees in the new healthcare environment. *Cambridge Quarterly of Healthcare Ethics, 6*, 299–301.

Crigger, B.-J. (1995). Negotiating the moral order: Paradoxes of ethics consultation. *Kennedy Institute of Ethics Journal, 5*(2), 89–112.

Crosthwaite, J. (1995). Moral expertise: A problem in the professional ethics of professional ethicists. *Bioethics, 9*, 361–379.

Degnin, F.D. (1997). Max Weber on ethics case consultation: A methodological critique of the conference on evaluation of ethics consultation. *The Journal of Clinical Ethics, 8,* 181–192.

Duval, G. (1997). Liability of ethics consultants: A case analysis. *Cambridge Quarterly of Healthcare Ethics, 6,* 269–281.

Edinger, W. (1992). Which opinion should a clinical ethicist give: Personal viewpoint or professional consensus? *Theoretical Medicine, 13,* 23-29.

Fink, A. (1993). *Evaluation fundamentals: Guiding health programs, research, and policy.* Newbury Park, CA: Sage.

Fletcher, J., & Siegler, M. (1996). What are the goals of ethics consultation? A consensus statement. *The Journal of Clinical Ethics, 7,* 122-126.

Fletcher, J.C. (1986). Goals and process of ethics consultation in health care. In J.F. Childress & R.D. Gaare (Eds.), *BioLaw* (Vol. II, pp. S:37–S:47). Frederick, MD: University Publications of America.

Fletcher, J.C. (1989). Standards for evaluation of ethics consultation. In J.C. Fletcher, N. Quist, & A.R. Jonsen (Eds.), *Ethics consultation in health care* (pp. 173–184). Ann Arbor, MI: Health Administration Press.

Fletcher, J.C. (1997). Ethics consultation and surrogates: Can we do better? *The Journal of Clinical Ethics, 8,* 50–59.

Fletcher, J.C., & Spencer, E.M. (1997). Ethics services in health care organizations. In J.C. Fletcher, P.A. Lombardo, M.F. Marshall, & F.G. Miller (Eds.), *Introduction to clinical ethics* (pp. 257–285). Frederick, MD: University Publishing Group.

Fox, E. (1996). Concepts in evaluation applied to ethics consultation research. *The Journal of Clinical Ethics, 7*(2), 116–121.

Fox, E., & Arnold, R.M. (1996). Evaluating outcomes in ethics consultation research. *The Journal of Clinical Ethics, 7,* 127–138.

Fox, E., & Tulsky, J.A. (1996). Evaluation research and the future of ethics consultation. *The Journal of Clinical Ethics, 7*(2), 146–149.

Fox, R.C. (1996). More than bioethics. *Hastings Center Report, 26*(6), 5–7.

Frader, J.E. (1992). Political and interpersonal aspects of ethics consultation. *Theoretical Medicine, 13,* 31–44.

Glover, J.J., Ozar, D.T., & Thomasma, D.C. (1986). Teaching ethics on rounds: The ethicist as teacher, consultant, and decision-maker. *Theoretical Medicine, 7,* 13–32.

Hoffman, P. (1996). Hospital mergers and acquisitions: A new catalyst for examining organizational ethics. *Bioethics Forum, 12*(2), 45–58.

Howe, E.G. (1996). The three deadly sins of ethics consultation. *The Journal of Clinical Ethics, 7,* 99–108.

Jonsen, A.R. (1980). Can an ethicist be a consultant? In V. Abernethy (Ed.), *Frontiers in medical ethics: Applications in a medical setting* (pp. 157–171). Cambridge, MA: Ballinger.

Jonsen, A.R. (1989). Mrs. Moore and the doctor of philosophy. In J.C. Fletcher, N. Quist, & A.R. Jonsen (Eds.), *Ethics consultation in health care* (pp. 149–154). Ann Arbor, MI: Health Administration Press.

Jonsen, A.R. (1993). Scofield as Socrates. *Cambridge Quarterly of Healthcare Ethics, 2,* 434–438.

Jonsen, A.R. (1996). Bioethics, whose crowd, and what ideology? *Hastings Center Report, 26*(6), 4–5.

Kaufert, J.M., & Putsch, R.W. (1997). Communication through interpreters in healthcare: Ethical dilemmas arising from differences in class, culture, language, and power. *The Journal of Clinical Ethics, 8,* 71-87.

Kelly, S.E., Marshall, P.A., Sanders, L.M., Raffin, T.A., & Koenig, B.A. (1997). Understanding the practice of ethics consultation: Results of an ethnographic multi-site study. *The Journal of Clinical Ethics, 8,* 136–149.

King, N.M.P. (1996). The ethics committee as Greek chorus. *HEC Forum, 8,* 346–354.

Kotin, A.M. (1996). Do no harm. *Bioethics Forum, 12*(2), 21–26.

La Puma, J., & Schiedermayer, D.L. (1991). The clinical ethicist at the bedside. *Theoretical Medicine, 12,* 141–149.

La Puma, J., & Schiedermayer, D.L. (1991). Ethics consultation: Skills, roles, and training. *Annals of Internal Medicine, 114*(2), 155–160.

La Puma, J., & Schiedermayer, D. (1994). *Ethics consultation: A practical guide.* Boston: Jones and Bartlett.

La Puma, J., & Toulmin, S.E. (1989). Ethics consultants and ethics committees. *Archives of Internal Medicine, 149,* 1109–1112.

Larkin, G.L., Adams, J.G., Derse, A.R., Iserson, K.V., & Gotthold, W.E. (1996). Managed care ethics: An emergency? *Annals of Emergency Medicine, 28,* 683–689.

Leeman, C.P., Fletcher, J.C., Spencer, E.M., & Fry-Revere, S. (1997). Quality control for hospitals' clinical ethics services: Proposed standards. *Cambridge Quarterly of Healthcare Ethics, 6,* 257–268.

Lilje, C. (1993). Ethics consultation: A dangerous, antidemocratic charlatanry? *Cambridge Quarterly of Healthcare Ethics, 2,* 438–442.

Lipkin, M., Putnam, S.M., & Lazare, A. (Eds.) (1995). *The medical interview: Clinical care education and research, frontiers of primary care.* New York: Springer.

Lusky, R.A. (1996). Educating healthcare ethics committees (EHEC) 1992–1996: The evaluation results. *HEC Forum, 8*(5), 247–289.

Lynch, A. (1994). . . . Has knowledge of [interpersonal] facilitation techniques and theory; has the ability to facilitate [interpersonally] . . . : fact or fiction? In F.E. Baylis (Ed.), *The health care ethics consultant* (pp. 45–62). Totowa, NJ: Humana Press.

Marsh, F.H. (1992). Why physicians should not do ethics consults. *Theoretical Medicine, 13,* 285–292.

Moreno, J.D. (1991). Call me doctor? Confessions of a hospital philosopher. *Journal of Medical Humanities, 12*(4), 183–196.

Moreno, J.D. (1991). Ethics consultation as moral engagement. *Bioethics, 5*(1), 44–56.

Moreno, J.D. (1996). Is ethics consultation an elegant distraction? *HEC Forum, 8*(1), 12–21.

Morreim, E.H. (1986). Philosophy lessons from the clinical setting: Seven sayings that used to annoy me. *Theoretical Medicine, 7,* 47–63.

Orr, R.D., Morton, K.R., deLeon, D.M., & Fals, J.C. (1996). Evaluation of an ethics consultation service: Patient and family perspective. *The American Journal of Medicine, 101,* 135–141.

Patton, M.Q. (1987). *How to use qualitative methods in evaluation.* Newbury Park, CA: Sage.

Pellegrino, E.D. (1988). Clinical ethics: Biomedical ethics at the bedside. *JAMA, 260,* 837–839.

Pellegrino, E.D., Siegler, M., & Singer, P.A. (1991). Future directions in clinical ethics. *Journal of Clinical Ethics, 2,* 5–9.

Potter, R.L. (1996). From clinical ethics to organizational ethics: The second stage of the evolution of bioethics. *Bioethics Forum, 12*(2), 3–12.

Potter, V.R. (1996). Individuals bear responsibility. *Bioethics Forum, 12*(2), 27–28.

Purtilo, R.B. (1989). A comment on the concept of consultation. In J.C. Fletcher, N. Quist, & A.R. Jonsen (Eds.), *Ethics consultation in health care* (pp. 99–108). Ann Arbor, MI: Health Administration Press.

Renz, D.O., & Eddy, W.B. (1996). Organizations, ethics, and health care: Building an ethics infrastructure for a new era. *Bioethics Forum, 12*(2), 29–39.

Rosner, F. (1997). The ethics of managed care. *The Mount Sinai Journal of Medicine, 64*(1), 8–19.

Ross, J.W. (1993). Why clinical ethics consultants might not want to be educators. *Cambridge Quarterly of Healthcare Ethics, 2,* 445–448.

Ross, J.W. (1996). Response to Jonathan Moreno [on ethics consultation]. *HEC Forum, 8*(1), 22–28.

Rubin, S., & Zoloth-Dorfman, L. (1996). She said/he said: Ethics consultation and the gendered discourse. *The Journal of Clinical Ethics, 7,* 321–332.

Schwartz, R.L., & Kushner, T. (1996). The role of institutional and community based ethics committees in the debate on euthanasia and physician-assisted suicide. *Cambridge Quarterly of Healthcare Ethics, 5,* 121–130.

Schyve, P.M. (1996). Patient rights and organization ethics: The Joint Commission perspective. *Bioethics Forum, 12*(2), 13–20.

Scofield, G.R. (1993). Ethics consultation: The least dangerous profession? *Cambridge Quarterly of Healthcare Ethics, 2,* 417–426.

Scofield, G.R. (1993). Here come the ethicists! *Trends in Health Care, Law and Ethics, 8*(4), 19–22.

Scofield, G.R. (1994). Ethics consultants, architects, and moral enclosures. *Trends in Health Care, Law and Ethics, 9*(4), 7–12.

Scofield, G.R. (1995). Ethics consultation: The most dangerous profession, a reply to critics. *Cambridge Quarterly of Healthcare Ethics, 4,* 225–228.

Self, D.J. (1993). Is ethics consultation dangerous? *Cambridge Quarterly of Healthcare Ethics, 2,* 442–445.

Self, D. J., & Skeel, J.D. (1986). Potential roles of the medical ethicist in the clinical setting. *Theoretical Medicine, 7,* 33–39.

Sexson, W.R., & Thigpen, J. (1996). Organization and function of a hospital ethics committee. *Clinics in Perinatology, 23,* 429–436.

Shapiro, R.S., Klein, J.P., & Tym, K.A. (1997). Wisconsin healthcare ethics committees. *Cambridge Quarterly of Healthcare Ethics, 6,* 288–292.

Siegler, M. (1992). Defining the goals of ethics consultations: A necessary step for improving quality. *QRB/Quality Review Bulletin, 18*(1), 15-16.

Siegler, M., Pellegrino, E.D., & Singer, P.A. (1990). Clinical medical ethics. *Journal of Clinical Ethics, 1,* 5–9.

Siegler, M., & Singer, P.A. (1988). Clinical ethics consultation: Godsend or God squad? *American Journal of Medicine, 85,* 759–760.

Singer, P.A., Pellegrino, E.D., & Siegler, M. (1990). Ethics committees and consultants. *Journal of Clinical Ethics, 1,* 263–267.

Skeel, J.D., & Self, D.J. (1989). An analysis of ethics consultation in the clinical setting. *Theoretical Medicine, 10*, 289–299.

Spencer, E.M. (1997). A new role for institutional ethics committees: Organizational ethics. *The Journal of Clinical Ethics, 8*, 372–376.

Thomasma, D.C. (1991). Why philosophers should offer ethics consultations. *Theoretical Medicine, 12*, 129–140.

Thomasma, D.C. (1993). Assessing bioethics today. *Cambridge Quarterly of Healthcare Ethics. 2*, 519–527.

Thornton, B., & Callahan, D. (1993). *Bioethics education: Expanding the circle of participants. A report of The Hastings Center on Bioethics Education.* Briarcliff Manor, NY: The Hastings Center.

Tulsky, J.A., & Fox, E. (1996). Evaluating ethics consultation: Framing the questions. *The Journal of Clinical Ethics, 7*, 109–115.

Tulsky, J.A., & Stocking, C.B. (1996). Obstacles and opportunities in the design of ethics consultation evaluation. *The Journal of Clinical Ethics, 7*, 139–145.

Veatch, R.M. (1989). Clinical ethics, applied ethics, and theory. In B. Hoffmaster, B. Freedman, & G. Fraser (Eds.), *Clinical ethics: Theory and practice.* Clifton, NJ: Humana Press.

Walker, M.U. (1993). Keeping moral spaces open: New images of ethics consulting. *Hastings Center Report, 23*(2), 33–40.

Weinstein, B.D. (1994). The possibility of ethical expertise. *Theoretical Medicine, 15*, 61–75.

West, M.B., & Gibson, J.M. (1992). Facilitating medical ethics case review: What ethics committees can learn from mediation and facilitation techniques. *Cambridge Quarterly of Healthcare Ethics, 1*, 63–74.

Whitley, E.M. (1996). A corporate approach to healthcare ethics. *Colorado Nurse, 96*(4), 30–32.

Wolf, S.M. (1991). Ethics committees and due process: Nesting rights in a community of caring. *Maryland Law Review, 50*, 798–858.

Yeo, M. (1993). Prolegomena to any future code of ethics for bioethicists. *Cambridge Quarterly of Healthcare Ethics, 2*, 403–415.

Zaner, R.M. (1993). Voices and time: The venture of clinical ethics. *Journal of Medicine and Philosophy, 18*(1), 9–31.

Zoloth-Dorfman, L., & Rubin, S.B. (1997). Navigators and captains: Expertise in clinical ethics consultation. *Theoretical Medicine, 18*, 421–432.

Index

Page numbers in *italics* denote tables.